KEY QUESTIONS IN

ANAESTHESIA

Second Edition

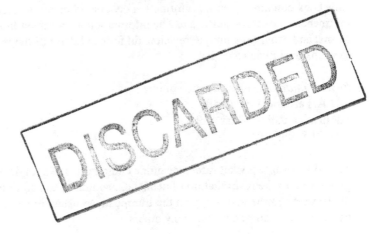

Also of interest:

Key Topics in Anaesthesia second edition
T.M. Craft and P.M. Upton
Publication date July 1995
ISBN 1 85996 075 8

This book contains essential information on a broad range of selected topics pertinent to modern anaesthesia. The information is presented in a problem-based format and provides a unique revision aid for candidates of the post-graduate examinations in anaesthesia.

Resuscitation: key data second edition
M.J.A. Parr and T.M. Craft
Publication date January 1995
ISBN 1 85996 060 X

An indispensable pocket reference guide containing essential data and treatment guidelines for the resuscitation of neonatal, paediatric, and adult patients. Includes the latest recommendations from the European Resuscitation Council, the American College of Surgeons and many others.

KEY QUESTIONS IN
ANAESTHESIA
Second Edition

T.M. Craft
MBBS FRCA
Consultant in Anaesthesia and Intensive Care,
Royal United Hospital, Bath, UK

P.M. Upton
MBBS MRCP(UK) FRCA
Consultant in Anaesthesia and Intensive Care,
Royal Cornwall Hospital, Treliske, Truro, UK

Provided by ZENECA Pharma as a service to medical education

βIOS
SCIENTIFIC
PUBLISHERS

©BIOS Scientific Publishers Limited, 1993, 1996

First published 1993 (ISBN 1 872748 52 X)
Second edition 1996 (ISBN 1 85996 220 3)

A CIP catalogue record for this book is available from the British Library.

ISBN 1 85996 220 3 (second edition)

BIOS Scientific Publishers Limited,
9 Newtec Place, Magdalen Road, Oxford OX4 1RE, UK.
Tel: +44 (0)1865 726286, Fax: +44 (0)1865 246823.
World Wide Web home page: http://www.Bookshop.co.uk/BIOS/

DISTRIBUTORS

Australia and New Zealand
　　DA Information Services
　　648 Whitehorse Road, Mitcham
　　Victoria 3132, Australia

India
　　Viva Books Private Ltd
　　4325/3 Anasari Road, Daryaganj
　　New Dehli 110002

Singapore and South East Asia
　　Toppan Company (S) PTE Ltd
　　38 Liu Fang Road, Jurong
　　Singapore 2262

USA and Canada
　　Books International Inc.
　　PO Box 605
　　Herndon VA 22070

Typeset by Els Boonen, BIOS Scientific Publishers Ltd, Oxford, UK.
Printed by Redwood Books, Trowbridge, UK.

This copy of *Key Questions in Anaesthesia second edition* is given as a service to medicine by ZENECA Pharma. Sponsorship of this copy does not imply the sponsors agreement or otherwise with the views expressed herein.

CONTENTS

ABBREVIATIONS

ACTH	Adrenocorticotrophic hormone
ADH	Antidiuretic hormone
ARDS	Adult respiratory distress syndrome
ASA	American Society of Anesthesiologists
ASD	Atrial septal defect
BMI	Body mass index
BMR	Basal metabolic rate
CNS	Central nervous system
CPAP	Continuous positive airways pressure
CSF	Cerebrospinal fluid
CVA	Cerebrovascular accident
CVP	Central venous pressure
CXR	Chest X-ray
DIC	Disseminated intravascular coagulopathy
DVT	Deep venous thrombosis
ECG	Electrocardiogram
EEG	Electroencephalogram
FEV_1	Forced expired volume in 1 second
FiO_2	Fraction of inspired gas that is oxygen
FRC	Functional residual capacity
HbA	Haemoglobin A
HIV	Human immunodeficiency virus
ICP	Intracranial pressure
IOP	Intra-ocular pressure
IPPV	Intermittent positive pressure ventilation
ITU	Intensive therapy unit
IU	International unit
LVEDV	Left ventricular end diastolic volume
MABP	Mean arterial blood pressure
MAC	Minimum alveolar concentration
MAOI	Monoamine oxidase inhibitor
MEAC	Minimum effective analgesic concentration
MH	Malignant hyperpyrexia

$PaCO_2$	Pressure of carbon dioxide in arterial blood
PEEP	Positive end expiratory pressure
PEFR	Peak expiratory flow rate
SDD	Selective decontamination of the digestive tract
SIRS	Systemic inflammatory response syndrome
SVC	Superior vena cava
TENS	Transcutaneous electrical nerve stimulation
TURP	Transurethral resection of the prostate
V:Q	Ventilation to perfusion ratio
VSD	Ventricular septal defect

PREFACE
to the second edition

Anaesthetic training in the UK is undergoing considerable change. This includes the examination for Fellowship of the Royal College of Anaesthetists which is scheduled to move from a three part to a two part examination. This will occur over a transitional period between late 1996 and 1998. Despite the change in the structure of the examination, the clinical approach of *Key Topics in Anaesthesia second edition* and the multiple choice questions contained within this book will remain relevant to the examination candidate.

Timothy M. Craft
Paul M. Upton

PREFACE
to the first edition

Multiple choice questions are now a component of many examinations including all three parts of the examination for Fellowship of the Royal College of Anaesthetists. Candidates sometimes attempt to create formulae or plans for answering MCQs but there is no substitute for practice.

This text comprises 360 multiple choice questions divided into four 'papers' of 90 questions each. This reflects the current arrangements in the Fellowship exam where the candidate is presented with 90 questions to answer in three hours. The reader is encouraged to approach the papers in exam-like conditions. An attempt should be made to answer the questions within strict time limits to not only provide practice at answering MCQs but also working at a rate which realistically represents that which is required by the exam. Each 'paper' of 90 questions should be allowed three hours for completion.

Anaesthesia is not an exact science with clear cut right or wrong answers to every problem. If you search hard enough you will find an exception to almost every rule. This should not be the approach to multiple choice questions. The examiners are not trying to trick you and efforts are made to ensure that questions are not ambiguous. Take the questions at face value and do not waste time looking for the catch. If you do not immediately know the answer, work from first principles and back your hunches; you will be right more often than you are wrong. The exam is 'negatively marked'; a wrong answer attracts a score of -1, wild guesses should thus be avoided.

Answers to the questions are provided at the back of the book with brief explanations where needed. The reader is referred to the appropriate pages in *Key Topics in Anaesthesia second edition* for a background to the question and its answers.

Working towards a common goal such as an examination with colleagues attempting to achieve the same end can be stimulating and enlightening. It is hoped that these questions and their answers will prompt thought and discussion leading to a better understanding of the subject.

Finally, if you feel that the answer given to any particular stem in this book is incorrect, please do not hesitate to let us know.

Timothy M. Craft
Paul M. Upton

PRACTICE PAPER ONE

Allow 3 hours for the completion of all 90 questions
Answers are on page 85

1.1 Pyloric stenosis may cause

A visible gastric peristalsis
B a hyperchloraemic alkalosis
C acid urine
D hypoventilation
E an increased risk of aspiration

1.2 Cardioplegia

A is used to stop the heart in systole
B usually contains approximately 30 mmol/l of potassium
C usually contains a membrane stabiliser such as procaine
D is cooled to 15°C prior to use
E results in a systemic fluid and electrolyte disturbance

1.3 Spinal opioids

A produce a more selective nocioceptive block than local anaesthetic agents
B act predominantly within the dorsal horn of the spinal cord
C are eliminated from the CSF by metabolism
D are associated with a high incidence of itching
E do not cause ventilatory depression beyond 6 hours after administration

1.4 Spinal anaesthesia

A may necessitate the administration of methoxamine, an alpha and beta agonist
B results in a lower incidence of post-dural puncture headache if pencil point needles are used
C should be accompanied by the administration of supplementary oxygen
D is likely to be more extensive if barbotage is used
E increases the incidence of postoperative urinary retention compared with general anaesthesia

1.5   Regarding gas scavenging

A   a canister of activated charcoal placed in the expiratory limb of a breathing system reliably absorbs nitrous oxide
B   the major component of soda lime is calcium hydroxide
C   anaesthetic gases may cause infertility in the partners of male anaesthetic staff
D   passive scavenging systems require a reservoir bag
E   passive scavenging systems do not require a negative pressure safety valve

1.6   Total parenteral nutrition is usually

A   isotonic when prepared as a mixed composite bag
B   comprised of 50 kcal of energy for every gram of nitrogen
C   provided with an energy source of 33% lipid and 67% carbohydrate
D   monitored by daily measurements of zinc, magnesium, and iron
E   provided in excess of the patient's metabolic requirements for the first week or so of feeding

1.7   The following are correct formulae for paediatric use

A   tracheal tube size (mm) after 1 year of age = (age x 0.5) + 4
B   tracheal tube length (cm) after 1 year of age = (age x 0.25) + 12
C   daily fluid requirement of a child weighing 20 kg = ~100 ml/kg/day
D   blood volume at birth = ~85 ml/kg
E   tissue oxygen requirement in a neonate = ~6 ml/kg/min

1.8   Phaeochromocytomata

A   are associated with medullary thyroid carcinoma
B   are associated with neurofibromatosis
C   are associated with multiple polyposis coli
D   occur outside the adrenal gland in ~10% of cases
E   are usually associated with pituitary hyperplasia

1.9   Ketamine

A   may stimulate opioid receptors
B   is contraindicated in those with glaucoma
C   is contraindicated in those with epilepsy
D   is associated with a high incidence of nausea and vomiting
E   sensitises the heart to catecholamines

1.10 A phaeochromocytoma

A may present with paroxysmal hypertension
B may secrete noradrenaline
C is a surgical emergency which should be operated on within 24 hours of the diagnosis being made
D may necessitate the use of intravenous phenoxybenzamine
E is usually associated with volume overload at presentation

1.11 Adverse drug reactions during anaesthesia

A depend on complement activation for the release of histamine
B usually result from the binding of circulating antibodies even if it is the patient's first anaesthetic
C are mediated by IgG in the case of immediate (type 1) reactions
D may be related to a genetic predisposition
E should be followed up by referral to the patient's GP for intradermal testing to establish the cause

1.12 The following are likely clinical problems during the perioperative care of a patient with Cushing's disease

A polycythaemia
B a low intravascular volume
C hyperkalaemia
D hypoglycaemia
E hyperpyrexia

1.13 Immediately following major surgery

A cortisol levels increase to up to ten times the preoperative level
B a decrease in peripheral vascular resistance is caused by cortisol
C hyperglycaemia may occur
D the stress response results in immunosuppression
E growth hormone is released from the adrenal glands

1.14 A patient with chronic bronchitis who retains CO_2 may exhibit

A a high V:Q ratio
B hypoxaemia
C cor pulmonale secondary to hypoxic pulmonary vasoconstriction
D an FEV_1:FVC ratio of 80%
E renal failure

1.15 Cardiac arrhythmias may occur with

A cardiomyopathy
B a low intracranial pressure
C phaeochromocytoma
D air emboli
E pneumothorax

1.16 The following are absolute indications for a double lumen tracheal tube

A resection of a bronchiectatic segment
B anterior spinal surgery
C oesophageal resection
D repair of a bronchopleural fistula
E resection of a giant lung cyst

1.17 With regard to tests supportive of brain death

A direct pupillary responses are absent but consensual reaction may be seen
B pupillary responses test the 2nd cranial nerve
C the corneal reflex tests the 3rd and 5th cranial nerves
D caloric testing results in nystagmus being seen
E doll's eyes movement means the eyes remain looking at a fixed point when the head is moved

1.18 The following statements are correct

A in a Bourdon pressure gauge an increase in pressure causes a curved tube to straighten
B flowmeters demonstrate turbulent flow at low flows
C the notch in the bobbin of a flowmeter is required to 'balance' the bobbin
D a pressure relief valve on the backbar protects the patient from barotrauma
E the oxygen failure device usually incorporates a mechanism to divert nitrous oxide to the atmosphere rather than the breathing system

1.19 The Jackson-Rees modification of Ayre's 'T'-piece

A is a low deadspace breathing system with a low resistance valve
B requires a fresh gas flow of 200 ml/kg/min (with a minimum of 3 l/min) when used for positive pressure ventilation
C requires a fresh gas flow of twice the minute ventilation when used for spontaneous ventilation
D has the advantage over Ayre's original 'T'-piece of humidifying the fresh gas
E cannot be used in children over 20 kg weight

1.20 With regard to the stress response to anaesthesia and surgery

A the anaesthetic is responsible for 30% of the response while surgery accounts for 70%
B preoperative morphine attenuates the stress response into the post-operative period
C cortisol release may be reduced using alpha and beta adrenoreceptor blockade
D the stress response is suppressed in paraplegic patients
E the obtunding effects of an epidural persist even when the sensory block has worn off

1.21 The following are associated with dystrophia myotonica

A cardiomyopathy
B renal failure
C predominant muscle wasting of the sternomastoids
D gonadal atrophy
E death in the fourth decade of life

1.22 Applied physics:

A the Coanda effect describes the attraction of a substance to the walls of the tube through which it is flowing
B Avagadro's number is the number of atoms in 1 g of carbon
C at room temperature one mole of gas occupies 22.4 litres
D Graham's law states that the rate of diffusion of a gas across a membrane is inversely proportional to the square root of its molecular weight
E after two time constants 95% of a process would have been completed if the initial rate of change had continued

1.23 **Following a perforating eye injury**

A surgery must be performed within the first four hours
B administration of suxamethonium results in a rise in intraocular pressure for 15 minutes
C a rapid sequence induction using a non-depolarising muscle relaxant may be indicated
D an empty stomach can only be guaranteed by waiting for at least 8 hours after the injury
E vitreous extrusion is relatively unimportant as it will regenerate

1.24 **Oxygen**

A is not flammable
B has a critical temperature of -85°C
C is produced commercially by distilling air
D is stored in the UK in black cylinders with white shoulders
E is stored in the UK in cylinders at a pressure of about 137 bar (~13 700 kPa) when full

1.25 **There is an increased risk of aspiration of gastric contents during anaesthesia in the following conditions**

A carcinoid syndrome
B diabetes mellitus
C dystrophia myotonica
D rheumatoid arthritis
E myasthenia gravis

1.26 **A gastroschiasis**

A is often associated with congenital cardiac defects
B usually necessitates an awake intubation
C places a neonate at particular risk from sepsis
D can result in bowel ischaemia following repair
E can be placed in a silastic sac and wound back into the abdomen over a few days

1.27 During cardiopulmonary resuscitation of a neonate

A external cardiac massage is performed using two fingers
B external cardiac massage is performed with a compression rate of 120/ minute (two/second)
C a single breath is given to every three compressions
D cardiac arrest is usually secondary to hypoxia
E initial defibrillation should be at 2 J/kg

1.28 Autonomic hyperreflexia following cervical cord transection

A may cause a hypertensive crisis
B may result in pulmonary impairment
C can be treated with ganglion blocking agents
D is associated with bradycardia
E will be moderated by volatile agents or regional anaesthesia

1.29 The incidence of perioperative deep venous thrombosis

A is approximately 25% amongst all surgical patients
B is reduced in women taking the combined oral contraceptive pill if it is stopped 3-4 weeks before major surgery
C is reduced in patients with left ventricular failure
D is higher in patients who have had a stroke
E is higher in patients who are septicaemic

1.30 Guillain-Barré syndrome

A usually starts one month after a viral illness
B may start with cranial nerve involvement
C causes a low CSF protein
D has a mortality rate of approximately 5%
E may be treated with plasmapheresis

1.31 An electrical current

A flows more readily through wet skin than dry skin
B is likely to cause muscle contraction when more than 100 mA is applied externally
C may be transmitted directly to the myocardium via a correctly functioning intracardiac catheter if it is connected to an earthed monitor
D is more likely to cause burns when it is transmitted to a large surface area of skin
E is less likely to be generated in a humid environment

1.32   With regard to high frequency ventilation

A   high frequency positive pressure ventilation may be performed using conventional tracheal tubes
B   expiration is passive during high frequency jet ventilation
C   expiration is active during high frequency oscillation
D   high frequency jet ventilators behave as constant flow generators
E   high frequency jet ventilation requires tidal volumes of ~5 ml/kg to maintain normocarbia

1.33   When compared with regional anaesthesia for transurethral resection of the prostate (TURP), general anaesthesia

A   makes bladder perforation easier to recognise
B   reduces the incidence of DVT
C   suppresses coughing
D   results in less blood loss
E   reduces the need for postoperative continuous bladder irrigation

1.34   Head injuries

A   account for 10% of deaths associated with road traffic accidents in Western Europe
B   necessitate admission to hospital in 25% of those attending Accident and Emergency departments following such an injury
C   when severe, are associated with hypoxaemia at the time of arrival in hospital in 85% of patients
D   are associated with a lucid interval following the initial trauma in up to 75% of patients who later die in the post-injury period
E   produce secondary brain damage as a result of cerebral ischaemia and hypoxaemia

1.35   Alveolar hypoventilation in a head injured patient may commonly result from

A   the initial trauma
B   the development of cerebral acidosis
C   unrelieved airway obstruction
D   the administration of mannitol
E   hyponatraemia

1.36 Sickle cell disease

A is inherited as an X-linked recessive disorder
B can be found in people of Mediterranean origin
C provides near complete protection against falciparum malaria
D can coexist with other haemoglobinopathies
E usually presents within the first month of life

1.37 In the history of anaesthesia

A the first widely witnessed ether anaesthetic for a surgical procedure in Europe was given in 1826
B nitrous oxide first became available in cylinders in the UK in 1868
C halothane was synthesised in 1937
D neuromuscular blockade was first used in clinical practice in 1942
E the local analgesic properties of conjunctival cocaine were described by Koller in 1884

1.38 Isoflurane

A has a MAC value of 0.75% in adults
B causes paroxysmal epileptiform spike activity on the EEG at concentrations greater than 3%
C has a blood:gas solubility at 37°C of 1.4
D increases the production of oral secretions
E is stored with added thymol as a stabiliser

1.39 The following should be omitted from the inspired gas mixture of a patient undergoing laser surgery to the upper airway

A nitrogen
B nitrous oxide
C helium
D humidification
E isoflurane

1.40 Sterilization may be achieved using

A 2% glutaraldehyde for 1 hour
B ethylene oxide
C dry heating
D steam at atmospheric pressure
E gamma irradiation

1.41 Hypothermia may be caused by

A increased conductive heat loss if the air temperature is low
B volatile agents which reset hypothalamic control to a lower 'normal'
C regional anaesthesia
D the use of humidified rather than unhumidified gases
E narcotic agents

1.42 Tetanus may cause

A myocarditis
B opisthotonos
C dysphagia
D psychosis
E life-long immunity following an acute attack

1.43 Patients with sickle cell disease presenting for anaesthesia

A should be maintained relatively hypovolaemic to decrease the risk of ARDS
B have an increased risk of infection
C should not receive regional anaesthesia such as a subarachnoid block
D should receive a normal inspired oxygen concentration
E should be transfused preoperatively to a haemoglobin concentration of >10 g/dl with a HbA concentration >40%

1.44 The sitting position

A is used in neurosurgery to the parietal lobes
B has a high risk of air embolism
C may necessitate the use of compression leggings
D can cause serious cerebral hypoperfusion
E results in worsening ventilation:perfusion mismatch when compared with the supine position

1.45 Acute systemic attacks of porphyria

A may be precipitated by pyrexia
B are unlikely if pancuronium is used as the muscle relaxant
C are painful, often requiring opioids
D occur in patients with abnormal haemoprotein production
E occur in porphyria cutanea tarda

1.46   Motor neurone disease

  A   may have a familial link
  B   can present with dysphagia
  C   has lower motor neurone symptoms which classically present in the legs
  D   is diagnosed by muscle biopsy and histological examination
  E   exhibits a normal sensitivity to non-depolarising muscle relaxants

1.47   Pulmonary oedema

  A   may present with orthopnoea
  B   can cause blood-tinged sputum
  C   does not impair gas exchange until marked symptoms have occurred
  D   results in an increase in pulmonary compliance
  E   classically causes fine expiratory crackles on auscultation

1.48   The findings during a thyrotoxic crisis may include

  A   delirium
  B   ketosis
  C   initial hypotension
  D   hypothermia
  E   abdominal pain

1.49   Infective endocarditis

  A   is most commonly caused by *Streptococcus faecalis*
  B   may result in cerebral abscess formation
  C   requires antibiotic cover for life
  D   may be prevented by giving amoxycillin orally
  E   should not be surgically treated in the acute illness as replacement valves always become infected

1.50   Tracheostomy

  A   may be performed under local anaesthesia
  B   tubes are initially changed on alternate days following operation
  C   tube cuff pressure should be maintained above 20 mmHg
  D   negates the need to humidify gases
  E   should be preceded with a sedative and antisialagogue premedicant

1.51 Volume overload during transurethral resection of the prostate (TURP) may result in

A headache
B hypotension
C bradycardia
D the need for CVP monitoring
E pulmonary infarction

1.52 Disadvantages of high frequency ventilation by comparison with conventional ventilation include

A increased cardiovascular instability
B increased mean airway pressure
C significant changes in tidal volume with changes in respiratory compliance
D difficulty with humidification of inspired gases
E inadequate ventilation when there is a disrupted airway (e.g. broncho-pleural fistula)

1.53 Aortic regurgitation

A may occur with a history of syphilis
B is associated with seropositive arthropathies
C may result in a quiet second heart sound
D can cause a systolic murmur
E may cause an Austin Flint diastolic murmur

1.54 Vomiting may cause

A pain
B the Mallory-Weiss syndrome
C hyperkalaemic alkalosis
D a fall in the intraocular pressure related to parasympathetic activity
E an increase in the pyloric sphincter tone

1.55 When monitoring inhaled agents

A photoacoustic spectrometry does not need the agent to be specified before measurement
B chemiluminescence may be used to measure nitric oxide
C mass spectrometry initially bombards the sample gas with electrons
D infrared absorption spectrometry has a slow response time
E the absorption into silicone rubber may be used

1.56 Air embolism may be diagnosed using

A 'basic senses'

B precordial auscultation to detect a machinery murmur

C capnography where a sudden rise in end expiratory CO_2 is seen

D a pulmonary artery catheter

E a Doppler ultrasound in the presence of as little as 0.5 ml of intravascular air

1.57 Babies with an inguinal hernia

A are usually born at term, but with a low birth weight

B always require at least a 2 day hospital admission for hernia repair

C may be anaesthetised using a laryngeal mask airway to control the airway

D have an increased risk of opioid sensitivity causing apnoea

E may present acutely with a strangulated hernia

1.58 The activated clotting time

A predominantly tests the intrinsic pathway

B is 'activated' with diatomaceous earth

C has a normal of approximately 100 seconds

D is difficult to perform in the operating theatre

E is unaffected by small doses of heparin (5000 i.u. intravenously)

1.59 Massive transfusion causes

A the oxygen dissociation curve to shift to the right with temperature change related to the transfusion

B clotting dysfunction related to temperature if the blood is <33°C

C the oxygen dissociation curve to shift to the left with the 2,3-DPG levels found in stored blood

D no change in albumin levels

E a low plasma ionised calcium which routinely warrants the administration of calcium

1.60 Central venous pressure

A measures blood volume
B has a 'c' wave which reflects isometric ventricular contraction against a closed tricuspid valve
C reflects right atrial pressure
D reflects venous capacitance
E monitoring increases the risk of air embolism

1.61 If a seizure occurs peroperatively

A further investigation is always necessary
B 'light' anaesthesia may be responsible
C the patient should be intubated immediately
D low potassium may be the cause
E hypothermia is a likely aetiology

1.62 Patient complications when using a direct arterial pressure monitor

A are more likely if hyperlipidaemia is present
B include central air embolism
C are related to the length of time an arterial cannula is in situ
D are reduced if Allen's test is used to assess radial artery blood flow
E are more likely if a non-compliant line is used to connect the cannula to the transducer

1.63 Autologous transfusion

A may be performed to reduce the risks of blood transfusion
B can be performed with predonation prior to emergency surgery
C can utilise the haemodilution technique
D with a predonation of up to 10 units is possible
E using a blood salvage technique is contraindicated if the patient requires cardiopulmonary bypass

1.64 A pulmonary artery catheter

A allows measurement of the cardiac index which is calculated as the cardiac output divided by the patient's weight
B requires X-ray screening for insertion
C always requires a thermistor at the tip of the catheter if cardiac output is to be measured
D allows direct measurement of the systemic vascular resistance
E may be used as a route of drug administration

1.65   In anaesthesia for elderly patients

A   hyoscine should be avoided as it causes respiratory depression
B   regional techniques result in greater hypotension than in younger patients
C   slow arm:brain circulation time has little clinical significance
D   IPPV is more likely to cause hypotension than in a younger patient
E   postoperative confusion is often related to hypoxia

1.66   The following may cause hyperpyrexia

A   endotoxins
B   atropine
C   humidifiers
D   thyrotoxicosis
E   an allergic reaction to drugs

1.67   With regard to the sensory supply of the upper airway

A   the anterior two-thirds of the tongue and the oropharynx are supplied by the glossopharyngeal nerve
B   the superior laryngeal nerve is a branch of the vagus nerve
C   the mucous membrane of the larynx below the rima glottidis is supplied by a branch of the recurrent laryngeal nerve
D   the cricothyroid membrane is supplied by the external branch of the superior laryngeal nerve
E   the hard and soft palate are supplied by the third division of the trigeminal nerve

1.68   Tracheal tubes considered safe for use with laser surgery to the airway

A   may be made of stainless steel
B   may be made of red rubber
C   may be made of plastic providing they are wrapped in adhesive aluminium foil
D   should have their cuffs filled with nitrous oxide
E   may have a cuff containing foam

1.69 **The following may exacerbate the weakness of well-controlled myasthenia gravis**

A hypokalaemia
B penicillin
C ciprofloxacin
D aminoglycosides
E edrophonium

1.70 **A chest X-ray should be performed during an acute asthmatic attack as**

A it will help assess the severity of the attack
B it may demonstrate a foreign body in the bronchial tree
C it may detect a pneumothorax
D it will allow severe narrowing of the large airways to be visualised
E atelectasis may be present

1.71 **Autoregulation of cerebral blood flow is impaired under the following conditions**

A hypertension
B hypoxia
C focal cerebral ischaemia
D seizure activity
E in the presence of a volatile anaesthetic agent

1.72 **Humidity may be measured**

A using a hair
B using a mass spectrometer
C using thermal conductivity techniques
D with a silver lined tube bathed in ether
E as the number of grams of water per unit volume of gas independent of temperature and pressure

1.73 **In a patient with a confirmed diagnosis of malignant hyperpyrexia the following are contraindicated**

A opioids
B propofol
C prophylactic dantrolene
D suxamethonium
E isoflurane

1.74 The following are recognised complications of hypotensive anaesthesia

A delayed wakening
B retraction ischaemia
C splenic infarction
D an increased incidence of DVT
E blindness

1.75 In a patient with hepatic dysfunction

A there is no alteration in the dose of thiopentone required to induce loss of consciousness
B coagulopathy resulting from thrombocytopenia occurs
C clearance of opioids is unaltered
D detoxification (hepatocellular) is frequently reduced but elimination (biliary) is rarely affected
E the FRC may be reduced

1.76 The Glasgow coma scale

A aims to document the depth of coma
B assesses eye opening on a 5-point scale
C gives a range of scores from 0-15
D indicates the need for ventilation if the score is <8
E assesses the best verbal response on a 5-point scale

1.77 In a patient with liver failure

A a high cardiac output (up to 14 l/min) may be seen
B dextrose/saline solutions should be used
C a metabolic acidosis is frequently seen
D lactulose is given as a laxative to clear the bowel
E neomycin may be given to 'sterilize' the bowel

1.78 Pre-eclampsia

A may result in placental failure and intrauterine death
B leads to vasospasm and hypovolaemia
C may cause haemorrhagic hepatic necrosis
D causes convulsions by altering cerebral electrolytes
E affects platelet function as well as platelet numbers

1.79 **The Apgar score**

A aims to assess the chances of a neonate developing normally after the first hour of life
B ranges from 0-12 points
C includes the assessment of muscle tone
D assesses reflex movements
E is less predictive than neurobehavioural scoring

1.80 **During an anaesthetic given to a pregnant woman for an unrelated procedure**

A maternal hyperoxia will result in fetal hyperoxia
B fetal acidosis may result from maternal vasodilation
C ketamine increases uterine tone
D light anaesthesia may be associated with fetal acidosis
E neostigmine may decrease uterine tone

1.81 **Pierre Robin syndrome**

A is related to cleft palate malformations
B may present with feeding difficulties
C causes severe symptoms which are maximal at 18 months of age
D may necessitate tracheostomy
E can cause heart failure

1.82 **Regional anaesthesia for Caesarean section**

A avoids the risk of maternal aspiration
B is strictly contraindicated in those with neurological disease
C may cause nausea
D may cause fixed dilated pupils (without death)
E can lead to the temporary development of a Horner's syndrome

1.83 **The following will prolong the duration of action of suxamethonium**

A ecothiopate
B cyclophosphamide
C isoflurane
D neostigmine
E morphine

1.84 Non-depolarising neuromuscular blockade may be potentiated by

A hyperthermia
B hypercalcaemia
C hypermagnesaemia
D dantrolene
E aminoglycosides - although this is a reversible phenomenon

1.85 The following may exacerbate diabetes mellitus

A the oral contraceptive pill
B spironolactone
C rifampicin
D hydrocortisone
E thiopentone

1.86 In diabetes mellitus

A the endocrine response to hypoglycaemia is reduced by anaesthesia
B the dose of premedicants should be reduced
C type II patients on oral medication always require insulin perioperatively
D unexpected cardiac arrest may occur more frequently than in non-diabetics
E β-blockade may make anaesthesia more dangerous

1.87 The signs of an acute exacerbation of asthma may include

A cough
B pulsus paradoxus where the systolic blood pressure rises by more than 10 mmHg on inspiration
C sweating
D no wheezing heard on chest auscultation
E fear

1.88 A patient with myasthenia gravis due to undergo thymectomy

A should have an intravenous cannula sited in a pedal vein
B may be expected to show a normal response to suxamethonium
C should have their anticholinesterase therapy increased in the immediate preoperative period
D may have a chronically elevated $PaCO_2$
E may complain of profound weakness following short periods of rest

1.89 **When anaesthetising patients with asthma**

A   a pressure controlled ventilator should be used
B   the I:E ratio is ideally set at 1:1
C   patients should routinely be extubated in a light plane of anaesthesia once protective airway reflexes have returned
D   intravenous theophyllines should be used at normal doses during anaesthesia
E   ketamine causes more bronchoconstriction than thiopentone

1.90 **The adult respiratory distress syndrome (ARDS) may result in**

A   cyanosis if the haemoglobin is 7 g/dl
B   alveolar oedema with a low protein content
C   possible evolution to an accelerated form of fibrosing alveolitis
D   denaturation of surfactant
E   the proliferation of type II alveolar cells

PRACTICE PAPER TWO

Allow 3 hours for the completion of all 90 questions
Answers are on page 95

2.1 Causes of peroperative hypertension include

A malignant hyperpyrexia
B stimulation of the carotid sinus
C hypocarbia
D drug interactions with monoamine oxidase inhibitors (MAOIs)
E the use of a blood pressure cuff which is too large

2.2 Obesity

A is always caused by a higher calorific intake than required
B may show differing distributions of adiposity
C is likely to be associated with the Pickwickian syndrome in 10% of morbidly obese patients
D is common in type I diabetes mellitus
E results in a decreased volume of distribution for fat soluble drugs

2.3 Dystrophia myotonica

A is inherited as an autosomal recessive disorder
B demonstrates anticipation (increasing severity in successive generations)
C has a preponderance of male sufferers
D causes hyperreflexia
E may result in muscle wasting

2.4 Intraocular pressure

A is independent of blood pressure
B may be affected by venous obstruction in the neck
C will be lowered by vasodilation in the presence of hypercarbia
D has a normal value of 16 mmHg
E is dependent on the drainage of aqueous humour and the vitreous volume

2.5 Inhaled anaesthetic agents

A may have their anaesthetic action reversed with high pressure
B probably act at the same site, as all agents have a similar molecular structure
C may exert their anaesthetic action by causing cell membrane expansion
D may exert their anaesthetic action by increasing lipid fluidity in the cell membranes
E also act at peripheral receptors in the nervous system

2.6 Regarding the gas laws

A Boyle's law states that at a constant temperature the volume of an ideal gas is inversely proportional to its pressure
B Charles' law states that at a constant volume the pressure of an ideal gas is proportional to its temperature
C the Ostwald solubility coefficient is related to standard temperature and pressure
D the Bunsen solubility coefficient is the volume of gas which dissolves in 1 unit volume of liquid at standard temperature and pressure where the partial pressure above the liquid is 1 atmosphere
E Dalton's law describes the total pressure exerted by a gas mixture

2.7 Patient controlled analgesia

A can be used as a research tool to compare equipotency between opioids
B is unsuitable for use for more than 1 week
C should use morphine whenever possible as this is the most suitable agent available
D may be of psychological benefit to a patient as they remain in control of their analgesia
E may be used to provide analgesia during labour

2.8 Tetralogy of Fallot

A has an ASD as part of the tetralogy
B is an acyanotic form of heart disease
C causes anaemia
D is associated with a 2nd heart sound with no splitting
E does not require cardiopulmonary bypass for a palliative systemic to pulmonary shunt to be inserted

2.9 Nitrous oxide

A is stored in blue cylinders with white shoulders in the UK
B is manufactured by heating ammonium nitrate
C is 35 times less soluble in blood than nitrogen
D may produce a megaloblastic anaemia following prolonged exposure
E counteracts the respiratory depressant effects of thiopentone at the induction of anaesthesia

2.10 When anaesthetising patients with permanent cardiac pacemakers

A depolarising muscle relaxants may lead to pacemaker inhibition
B volatile anaesthetic agents raise the stimulation threshold and may result in the loss of pacemaker capture
C a magnet placed over the patient's heart ensures that the pacemaker is in a fixed pacing mode
D isoprenaline is the drug of choice for the resuscitation of a patient without an intrinsic rhythm in the event of pacemaker failure
E the surgeon should be requested not to use bipolar diathermy

2.11 Myasthenia gravis

A is usually congenitally acquired
B is characterised by fatiguable muscle weakness
C results from a reduction in the number of functioning postsynaptic acetylcholine receptors at the neuromuscular junction
D occurs equally amongst men and women
E may be associated with autoimmune diseases

2.12 Acute epiglottitis

A may present with severe respiratory obstruction and necessitate an awake intubation
B usually presents with a floppy, exhausted child who wants to lie down and be left to sleep
C is best treated with penicillin and gentamicin until microbiological sensitivities are known
D does not occur in those aged over 16
E is an absolute indication for re-examination of the larynx under deep anaesthesia before extubation

2.13 Fat embolism

A only occurs following a fracture
B is associated with cerebral dysfunction
C may result in the development of ARDS
D may result in fat being seen in the urine, sputum or retinal blood vessels
E is a contraindication to fixation of the associated fracture

2.14 Anaemia

A is a common cause of a low saturation recorded by pulse oximeters during anaesthesia
B is associated with decreased tissue oxygen delivery when the haematocrit is 0.3
C is likely to be better tolerated during anaesthesia when it is caused by chronic renal failure than by an acute gastrointestinal haemorrhage
D may result in increased capillary blood flow
E in a healthy 3-month infant is defined as a haemoglobin <11 g/dl

2.15 The following instrumental techniques have been proposed for monitoring the depth of anaesthesia

A skin conductance
B rectal tone
C oesophageal contractility
D urinary bladder contractility
E electromyography of the frontalis muscle

2.16 Hyperaldosteronism

A usually results from the administration of exogenous hormones
B is a cause of hyperkalaemia
C is associated with respiratory muscle weakness
D causes hyperpigmentation
E is a contraindication to epidural anaesthesia

2.17 Etomidate

A is a phencyclidine derivative
B inhibits aldosterone responses to ACTH
C is presented in 35% propylene glycol
D is hydrolysed by circulating esterases
E has a pH of 10-11

2.18   **Adverse drug reactions during anaesthesia**

A   are usually related to the known pharmacological actions of a drug
B   may present with severe bronchospasm and hypotension
C   should be treated in the first instance with hydrocortisone and anti-histamines
D   may necessitate external cardiac compressions unless the patient is in sinus rhythm
E   should as a last resort be treated with repeated intravenous doses of adrenaline

2.19   **The diagnosis of brain death in the UK**

A   may be made in a self-ventilating patient provided that they can be shown to be in a chronic vegetative state
B   requires that the patient's temperature is greater than 36°C
C   must be confirmed by at least one EEG
D   cannot be made in the presence of a markedly elevated PaCO$_2$
E   cannot be made in the presence of severe hypotension

2.20   **When resuscitating patients with burns**

A   it is important to adhere strictly to a formula for the replacement of fluid
B   analgesic requirements are low as the burned area is usually insensitive
C   the patient should be kept exposed and cool in order to dissipate thermal energy
D   circumferential burns of the neck are an indication for early intubation
E   blood is rarely required but large clear fluid transfusions are common

2.21   **During cardiopulmonary resuscitation of an adult**

A   the correct rate for external cardiac massage is 60 compressions/ minute (1/second)
B   external cardiac massage is performed over the mid-point of the sternum
C   external cardiac massage should depress the sternum by 3-4 cm
D   a single rescuer should give 2 breaths every 15 compressions
E   with two rescuers a single breath should be given for every five compressions

2.22 **Carbon dioxide**

    A is colourless and has a pungent odour at high concentrations
    B is stored for clinical use as a gas in grey cylinders
    C produces a rise in CSF pH
    D reduces sympathetic vasomotor tone
    E stimulates respiration by acting directly on a respiratory centre in the floor of the fourth ventricle

2.23 **Patients with a higher risk of developing a perioperative deep venous thrombosis include**

    A those with cardiac failure
    B day case patients
    C smokers
    D those with a malignancy
    E those with sickle cell disease

2.24 **With regard to dental anaesthesia**

    A if general anaesthesia is being administered by a single-handed, operating dentist it is a legal requirement that he is trained in anaesthetic techniques
    B an infraorbital nerve block will anaesthetise the ipsilateral incisors
    C relative analgesia refers to the inhalation of 30% oxygen in nitrous oxide
    D incremental intravenous methohexitone may be used for dental sedation
    E it is recommended that dental patients who have received general anaesthesia should not drive a car for 6 hours

2.25 **Oxygen**

    A is a stable molecule with an indefinite half-life
    B may cause grand mal convulsions
    C may cause fibroplasia behind the retina of neonates
    D may cause fatal respiratory depression
    E is repelled by a magnetic field

2.26 **Complications of insertion of a pulmonary artery catheter include**

A endocarditis
B pulmonary infarction
C coronary sinus cannulation
D pulmonary vasodilation
E rupture of a pulmonary artery

2.27 **Regarding perioperative ECG monitoring**

A a V_5 lead will only detect 60% of ECG detectable ischaemic episodes
B a V_5 lead in combination with lead II will detect 96% of ischaemic episodes
C lead II is used if arrhythmias are anticipated
D multilead systems are required to detect ST segment depression
E acute electrolyte imbalance may be detected

2.28 **The following are widely regarded as contraindications to day surgery**

A the need to admit >1% of patients after a procedure
B a patient of 1 year of age
C the need to drive within 24 hours of a general anaesthetic
D the need for intubation
E ASA III/IV patients

2.29 **In the elderly**

A FRC is reduced but residual volume is unchanged with increasing age
B chest wall compliance is decreased
C closing volume exceeds FRC in patients over 45 years when standing
D there is a normal response to an elevated $PaCO_2$
E hepatic function decreases by 1% per year after 30 years of age

2.30 **Epilepsy**

A has an incidence of 1 in 200
B may necessitate the use of muscle relaxants to prevent metabolic acidosis
C may affect sensation
D may be psychomotor in nature
E is treated by raising the electrical threshold for seizure activity

2.31 Heat and moisture exchange devices

A are an example of active humidification
B can warm and humidify inspired gases to body temperature and 90% humidity
C utilise condensation of water from the expired gas
D result in increased dead space of a breathing system
E may cause burns to the airway

2.32 If a clinical diagnosis of malignant hyperpyrexia is made during a general anaesthetic

A the patient should have their FIO_2 increased to 0.5
B minute ventilation should remain the same so that the increased CO_2 production may be noted in order to confirm the diagnosis
C dantrolene is given (10 mg/kg i.v.) and repeated if necessary
D mannitol is contraindicated
E clotting studies are not indicated as they will be normal

2.33 With regard to patients with hypertension

A all such patients should preoperatively have their urea and electrolytes measured, and a chest X-ray and an ECG performed
B a β-adrenergic blocker given with the premedicant may help prevent perioperative myocardial ischaemia
C the preoperative plasma volume is normal
D systemic vascular resistance is elevated
E hypothermia is a recognised cause of postoperative hypertension

2.34 Deliberate hypotensive anaesthesia is contraindicated in

A hepatic dysfunction
B pregnancy
C resection of a parietal lobe glioma
D glaucoma when treated with ganglion blockers
E total hip replacement

2.35 Ankylosing spondylitis

A has an equal sex incidence
B is associated with HLA Bw18
C is related to apical fibrosing alveolitis
D is more frequently found in patients with aortic valve incompetence
E occurs more commonly in those patients who have an increased bowel frequency

2.36 Laryngectomy

A rarely results in large blood loss
B may cause peroperative bradycardia
C is a recognised 'risk' operation for the development of pneumothorax
D may result in air embolism
E is not an indication for hypotensive anaesthesia as patients are generally frail

2.37 Nitric oxide

A is delivered from a red cylinder
B is found in cigarette smoke
C only very rarely has nitrogen dioxide as a contaminant
D may cause methaemoglobinaemia
E is administered in the fresh gas flow in concentrations up to 200 parts per million

2.38 Halothane hepatitis

A may occur because 10% of halothane is metabolised
B may occur if the usual reductive metabolism of halothane changes to an alternative metabolic pathway
C has an incidence in children of approximately 1 in 80 000
D is most likely in obese, middle-aged men
E may occur after a single exposure

2.39 Pre-eclampsia

A occurs in 5% of pregnancies
B is more common in women who drink alcohol
C is commonest at 32 weeks gestation
D is diagnosed following the finding of the triad of hypertension, a low plasma albumin and oedema
E is more common in diabetic patients

2.40 APACHE scoring

A stands for accurate physiological and chronic health evaluation
B aims to predict outcome for an individual
C uses 12 physiological variables in the APACHE II system
D ignores the primary diagnosis as this has no bearing on outcome
E uses the best physiological values seen within 24 hours of admission

2.41 Regarding cardiac surgery

A either angiography or echocardiography is usually performed prior to elective surgery
B awareness is a particular risk during rewarming
C while on cardiopulmonary bypass there is no need to administer anaesthetic agents
D oxygen should not be given via the trachea whilst on bypass as it will confuse blood gas analysis for the bypass technician
E 1 mg of protamine will reverse 1 mg of heparin

2.42 In a patient with renal failure

A protein bound drugs have an increased free fraction
B lipid insoluble drugs are predominantly metabolised by the liver
C uraemia has no pharmacodynamic effects
D hypovolaemia is often present
E the standard bicarbonate is normal

2.43 The following are commonly used to treat supraventricular tachycardia

A lignocaine
B amiodarone
C DC shock
D adenosine
E carotid sinus massage

2.44 Sedation in the intensive care unit

A may be used to manage confusional states
B may decrease the psychological trauma of treatment
C can be well assessed using heart rate and blood pressure
D may impair the immune response
E can be used rather than analgesic agents postoperatively

2.45 During pregnancy

A the ECG may show left axis deviation with flattened/inverted T waves in lead III
B the peak cardiac output (30% above normal) is not reached until the 38th week
C IVC obstruction can occur from the 20th week
D stroke volume increases to a greater extent than heart rate
E brachial blood pressure accurately reflects uterine blood flow

2.46 The following are commonly thought to be teratogenic

A halothane
B noscapine
C folate
D vitamin A
E isoflurane

2.47 General anaesthesia for Caesarean section

A is associated with a higher maternal mortality rate than regional anaesthesia
B is preferred if placenta accreta is present
C should be preceded with at least 3 minutes of preoxygenation
D is associated with increased uterine bleeding if 0.75 MAC of a volatile agent is used
E results in identical neonatal 1 minute Apgar scores as in those neonates delivered by emergency Caesarean section under regional anaesthetic

2.48 Local anaesthetic toxicity

A may result in hypoxia
B may need treatment that includes thiopentone
C is treated with ephedrine
D causes tinnitus, perioral paraesthesia and fasciculations of the tongue
E is more likely with prilocaine rather than lignocaine

2.49 Suxamethonium (1 mg/kg)

A binds to acetylcholinesterase to prevent its action
B raises potassium by 0.5 mmol/l in a normal patient
C increases intragastric pressure
D does not affect oesophageal sphincter tone
E may increase jaw muscle tension

2.50 Regarding non-depolarising muscle relaxants

A train of four responses are equally depressed for each twitch
B post-tetanic counting is performed following a 50 Hz stimulus applied for 10 seconds
C a post-tetanic count of 6 implies the train of four response will begin to return within 10 minutes
D edrophonium has a more rapid onset of action than neostigmine
E the ability to perform a head lift for five seconds is an unreliable sign of adequate reversal

2.51 The following are important factors when considering gastric emptying after trauma

A pain
B prokinetic agents
C the administration of pethidine
D the length of time between the last meal and the time of trauma
E associated minor head injury

2.52 Diabetes

A has a prevalence of 1%
B is caused by the complete lack of endogenous insulin
C is associated with obesity
D may result in a decreased FEV_1 and FVC
E can cause microalbuminuria

2.53 Autonomic neuropathy is associated with

A ankle swelling
B orthostatic hypotension
C diarrhoea
D an increased heart rate response to a Valsalva manoeuvre
E delayed gastric emptying

2.54 **When checking an anaesthetic machine**

A the electrical supply, if present, should be disconnected
B a carbon dioxide cylinder should not be attached to the machine
C the oxygen analyser is calibrated only by the medical physics department
D -150 mmHg is adequate suction pressure
E using the oxygen flush will not cause a fall in the oxygen pipeline pressure

2.55 **Adult Respiratory Distress Syndrome (ARDS) is a diagnosis made using the following findings**

A a pulmonary artery wedge pressure of 20 mmHg or higher
B pulmonary infiltrates seen on the CXR
C high inflation pressures during ventilation
D a high respiratory compliance
E hypercarbia

2.56 **Anaemia results in**

A a left shift of the oxygen dissociation curve
B errors in pulse oximetry
C decreased buffering capacity for CO_2 induced pH changes
D a decreased urine output
E increased oxygen extraction

2.57 **Patients with pyloric stenosis should be operated on**

A after resuscitation with 5% dextrose
B before a nasogastric tube is inserted as it may otherwise perforate the distended stomach
C early if a secondary gastritis is suspected
D only when the bicarbonate is between 24 and 30 mmol/l
E following an awake intubation to prevent aspiration

2.58 **The Cardiff Aldasorber**

A is used to scavenge volatile agents
B results in a decreased incidence of spontaneous miscarriage in theatre staff when it is used regularly
C contains soda lime mixed with activated charcoal
D is discarded after 100 hours of use
E is not widely used due to its cost

2.59 **A spinal anaesthetic**

A may be complicated by transverse myelitis
B results in a better quality of block if hyperbaric rather than plain solutions are used
C may result in an extradural haematoma
D may be prolonged if vasoconstrictors are added
E is likely to cause bradycardia if the block reaches T_4

2.60 **The clinical signs of hypercarbia include**

A hypertension
B bradycardia
C cool, clammy peripheries
D miosis
E tremor

2.61 **Electrical diathermy**

A has a current frequency of 0.3-3 MHz
B has a lower frequency when used for cutting than when used for coagulation
C relies on a low current density for effective function
D may result in injury to the tracheal mucosa if the tracheal tube is earthed via the anaesthetic machine
E must be of the bipolar type if it is to be used within 25 cm of a flammable anaesthetic source

2.62 **The following are reliable indicators of malnutrition**

A arm circumference measurements
B a 24 hour urinary amino acid estimation
C weight loss
D hair loss
E serum albumin

2.63 **The following are typical indications for an awake intubation**

A severe respiratory failure
B severe coronary artery disease
C a full stomach
D upper airway obstruction
E raised intracranial pressure

2.64 **Oxygen desaturation is more likely in a child than an adult because**

A children have a higher oxygen requirement on a weight basis
B children have a higher metabolic rate
C children have an immature respiratory system
D adult haemoglobin binds more strongly to oxygen
E children have a low FRC

2.65 **Phaeochromocytomata**

A are chromaffin cell adrenocortical tumours
B may be familial
C have usually metastasised by the time the patient presents for surgery
D may be associated with postural hypotension
E may be found at the aortic bifurcation

2.66 **During general anaesthesia the functional residual capacity**

A may be a vital source of oxygen if there is difficulty with intubation at induction
B falls as a result of cranial displacement of the diaphragm
C is maintained providing muscle relaxants are not administered
D falls as a result of intra-abdominal vasodilatation
E is relatively maintained if ketamine is the anaesthetic agent used

2.67 **Coronary blood flow**

A is approximately 250 ml/min at rest
B results in a supply of haemoglobin which unloads a maximum of 50% of its oxygen
C is decreased if the diastolic blood pressure increases
D reduction may cause arrhythmias
E occurs mainly in systole when the aortic blood pressure is higher

2.68 **Methohexitone**

A is presented as a 10% solution
B is more potent than thiopentone
C exists in a non-ionised form at body pH to a greater extent than thiopentone
D results in less respiratory depression than thiopentone at equipotent doses
E crosses the blood-brain barrier less readily than thiopentone

2.69 When using high frequency oscillation

A the pattern of expiration is a mirror image of inspiration
B a bias gas flow is required to ensure removal of CO_2
C the stroke volume of the oscillator is usually less than the volume of the conducting airways
D the frequency of ventilation lies in the range 60-120 cycles per minute
E expiration is passive

2.70 The following are likely sequelae after a near-drowning

A pulmonary oedema
B cerebral oedema
C acute pancreatitis
D profound alkalosis
E renal failure

2.71 When considering the respiratory system of a child

A the angle of the carina is wider than that of an adult
B the number of alveolae in the lung is maximal shortly after birth
C the chest wall is less compliant than that of an adult
D the expiratory pause of a neonate is ~1 second
E there is less ventilation:perfusion mismatch than in adults

2.72 Neonates

A may revert to a transitional circulation if they are rendered hyperoxaemic
B have a blood volume of ~85 ml/kg
C have a normal haemoglobin of ~16 g/dl
D have a relatively fixed heart rate and usually increase their cardiac output by increasing stroke volume
E usually have a more muscular right ventricle than left ventricle

2.73 During the catabolic phase associated with the stress response to surgery

A ADH levels are unchanged
B prolactin levels are decreased
C the actions of insulin are suppressed
D noradrenaline is released to a greater extent than adrenaline
E cardiac contractility increases

2.74 During one lung ventilation

A the severity of shunt is affected by the severity of preoperative lung disease
B the same tidal volume is used as with two lung ventilation provided that the airway pressures are not excessive
C a minimum FIO_2 of 0.75 should be used
D CPAP may be applied to the unventilated lung
E PEEP of up to 10 cm of H_2O is usually beneficial in preventing hypoxaemia when applied to the ventilated lung

2.75 Rheumatoid arthritis may result in

A Caplan's syndrome
B mononeuritis multiplex
C spinal cord compression
D lower motor neurone lesions
E anaemia (usually macrocytic)

2.76 Sickle cell trait

A results in death usually in the 4th to 5th decade
B can be differentiated from the homozygote using a Sickledex test
C may result in sickling with mild hypoxaemia
D usually results in anaemia with a haemoglobin concentration of approximately 9 g/dl in adults
E is associated with an increased incidence of pulmonary infarction

2.77 Coarctation of the aorta

A is associated with Turners syndrome
B is commoner in females
C usually occurs proximal to the origin of the left subclavian artery
D may cause rib notching on the chest X-ray
E may be dilated using percutaneous balloon angioplasty

2.78 Decontamination of equipment

A results in the destruction of organisms but not spores
B is achieved by boiling
C is often performed prior to items being returned to a sterilisation department
D can be achieved by cleaning items by hand
E is sufficient to prevent cross contamination with hepatitis B virus

2.79 Suction apparatus for emergency anaesthetic use requires

A delivery tubing that is compliant
B a reservoir with a large capacity to permit the rapid development of a high negative pressure
C a catheter that is wide and short
D a gauge that displays negative pressure in a clockwise fashion
E a reservoir cut-off valve

2.80 Body temperature can be

A monitored accurately and without risk via the nasopharynx
B measured using a thermistor (where resistance changes linearly with temperature)
C measured using a thermocouple (where resistance rises with temperature)
D can be monitored via a urinary catheter
E can be assessed via the tympanic membrane which accurately reflects the brain temperature

2.81 An acute attack of tetanus

A may necessitate paralysis and ventilation for management of muscle spasms
B may be treated with β-blockers to prevent sympathetic overactivity
C results in worsening symptoms for ten days
D is diagnosed by culture of the causative organism
E is treated with benzyl penicillin and human tetanus immunoglobulin

2.82 Pressure necrosis occurring in theatre

A is more likely to occur on the lateral aspect of the lower limb when the lithotomy position is used
B is a particular risk in those with connective tissue disorders
C may occur following the use of an anaesthetic mask
D is more likely to occur on the heel than the elbow
E is less likely in the obese patient

2.83 Magnetic resonance imaging

A requires cryogenic magnets utilising helium at 4 degrees Kelvin
B does not interfere with pulse oximetry although ECG monitoring is difficult
C is easily performed in children as it is non invasive
D is very rapid taking a maximum of five minutes to image a patient
E is safe in patients with intrauterine contraceptive devices

2.84 The following may exacerbate the symptoms of multiple sclerosis

A cold
B stress
C exercise
D general anaesthesia
E regional anaesthesia

2.85 The following may precipitate an acute attack in a patient with acute intermittent porphyria

A neostigmine
B suxamethonium
C methohexitone
D bupivacaine
E halothane

2.86 The following are recognised complications of thyroid surgery

A tracheal oedema
B pneumothorax
C acute hypercalcaemia
D air embolism
E corneal ulceration

2.87 Mitral stenosis

A may be associated with presystolic accentuation of the first heart sound if the patient is in atrial fibrillation
B commonly causes haemoptysis and recurrent bronchitis
C results in a diastolic murmur, the duration of which is proportional to the severity of the stenosis
D may cause an opening snap and a loud first heart sound
E should be managed by ensuring that pulmonary vasodilation does not occur during anaesthesia

2.88 In major aortic surgery

A renal perfusion is well maintained provided that cross clamping is distal to the renal arteries
B myocardial strain is most likely when the cross clamp is released
C dopamine, mannitol and frusemide may all be used to preserve urine output in the hypoperfused kidney
D the fall in blood pressure when the cross clamp is released is solely related to the increased blood flow distal to the graft
E heparin (5000 i.u. intravenously) may need reversal

2.89 The following are suggestive of an air embolism in an 'at risk' patient

A coughing
B bradycardia
C jugular venous distention
D chest pain
E hypertension

2.90 Cross matching of blood

A determines the Rhesus group of the patient
B on just the ABO system results in a 3% chance of an incompatible transfusion per unit transfused
C with a full cross match achieves compatibility in 99.95% of cases
D should be performed prior to a femoral popliteal bypass
E in group AB Rhesus positive patients may be safely omitted as they are 'universal recipients'

PRACTICE PAPER THREE

Allow 3 hours for the completion of all 90 questions
Answers are on page 105

3.1 Blood filters

A found in blood giving sets have a pore size of up to 100 μm
B are used to remove microaggregates which occur particularly with red cell transfusions
C may stimulate histamine release
D may activate clotting mechanisms
E may lose efficiency if flow streaming occurs

3.2 The activated partial thromboplastin time

A tests the extrinsic pathway
B is dependent on clotting factors synthesised using vitamin K
C is prolonged if heparin is present
D has a normal result of 20-22 seconds
E is 'activated' by kaolin or cephaloplastin

3.3 Carcinoid tumours

A may secrete bradykinin
B arise from enterochromaffin cells
C may secrete histamine
D are most usually found as a primary tumour in the large bowel
E can result in pellagra

3.4 Ischaemic heart disease

A is most easily diagnosed with a 12 lead ECG
B may be treated with calcium antagonists
C means that isoflurane should not be used
D requires the preload to be high to minimise LVEDV and therefore oxygen demand
E is diagnosed by a raised CK(MB) isoenzyme

3.5 **Rheumatoid arthritis is associated with**

A amyloidosis
B the nephrotic syndrome
C focal epilepsy
D Sjögren's syndrome
E vasculitis

3.6 **A sickle cell crisis**

A occurs when cells are exposed to hypoxia or alkalosis
B results in initial reversible sickling which subsequently becomes irreversible
C has pain, caused by tissue hypoxia, as a predominant symptom
D can present with priapism
E may be a cause of transient ischaemic attacks

3.7 **Following an acute cervical cord transection**

A a CVA may occur
B gastric stasis commonly occurs
C residual lung volume is reduced
D it is mandatory to perform tracheal intubation using an awake fibreoptic technique
E Ondine's curse may occur

3.8 **Hypothermia results in**

A a risk of asystolic cardiac arrest below 28°C
B a decreased level of consciousness below 33°C
C decreased CO_2 production
D a decreased glomerular filtration rate and urine output below 28°C
E a decrease in MAC requirement of 15% per degree of temperature fall

3.9 **Tetanus**

A has an equal sex incidence
B alters excitatory synaptic function resulting in muscle rigidity
C is transmitted within the body by neural pathways
D has an incubation period of 2-45 days
E usually results in no residual deficit if the patient survives

3.10 The following may occur after positioning of the anaesthetised patient

A an increase in chest compliance
B retinal ischaemia and blindness from pressure to the eye
C a fall in the intracranial pressure
D increased surgical bleeding
E meralgia paraesthetica

3.11 Patients with variegate porphyria

A have aminolaevulinic acid in their urine
B have porphyrins in their faeces even when the disease is in a latent phase
C should be managed during an acute attack with carbohydrate loading, β-blockers and fluids
D have a deficiency of uroporphyrinogen-1-synthetase
E are often Scandinavian

3.12 Pulmonary oedema may

A be caused by a decreased capillary permeability such as occurs in fat embolism
B be caused by a rapid re-expansion of a lung following a pneumothorax
C be associated with acute brain injury
D be related to altitude
E occur if the usual lymphatic drainage of 100 ml per day is exceeded

3.13 Patients with congenital heart disease

A do not need prophylactic antibiotics if the abnormality does not involve the cardiac valves
B which is cyanotic should have their systemic vascular resistance increased
C may benefit from nitric oxide to lower the pulmonary vascular resistance
D with a right to left shunt have slower intravenous induction times than normal
E are at increased risk of cerebral air embolism if a left to right shunt occurs

3.14 The following may be associated with thyroid surgery for goitre

A venous obstruction
B rheumatoid arthritis
C tracheochondromalacia
D abnormal glucose tolerance
E myopathy

3.15 An MRI scanner

A has a 500 Gauss line drawn around it, outside of which ferromagnetic objects may be placed
B does not interfere with non invasive BP measurement
C may cause patient burns
D produces a magnetic field that is approximately 1000 times stronger than the earth's
E will suffer from image degradation if iron objects are near the scanner

3.16 The following are recognised early complications of tracheostomy

A erosion into the oesophagus
B pneumothorax
C cardiovascular collapse
D tracheal stenosis
E surgical emphysema

3.17 Glycine solution used for transurethral resection of the prostate (TURP)

A is hyperosmotic
B is a good electrical conductor and thus permits the use of diathermy
C has optical properties which prevent distortion of vision
D is absorbed at a rate of approximately 5 ml/min
E may result in CNS toxicity related to systemic glycine

3.18 Regarding postoperative vomiting

A metoclopramide has actions at both the chemoreceptor trigger zone and the vomiting centre

B butyrophenones work predominantly at the vomiting centre

C nitrous oxide is not likely to be causative provided that the patient has normal middle ears

D anticholinergic agents mainly exert their actions after crossing the blood-brain barrier

E methohexitone is more likely to be implicated than etomidate

3.19 Acquired immunodeficiency syndrome

A usually occurs after a 3 month window following infection with HIV

B results from preferential dysfunction of T killer cells

C may present with malignancy

D may be perinatally acquired

E is caused by a retrovirus

3.20 As part of the management of peroperative air embolism

A the surgeon should immediately flood the wound with saline

B N_2O is discontinued as it is 44 times more soluble in blood than nitrogen

C the patient's neck should be compressed if a neurosurgical cause is suspected

D a central line placed in the SVC can be used to aspirate air

E the right lateral head down position will trap air in the right ventricle

3.21 Storage of blood

A is optimal at 2°C

B should permit a minimum of 95% of cells to be viable 24 hours after transfusion

C with sodium chloride, adenine, glucose and mannitol provides a shelf life of 45 days

D with citrate, phosphate and dextrose provides a shelf life of 35 days

E may be performed in a frozen state with glycol

3.22 The prothrombin time

A tests the intrinsic pathway
B tests the pathway that utilises the vitamin K dependent factors XII, XI, IX and VIII
C is the first coagulation test to be affected by warfarin
D has a normal result of 12-14 seconds
E is 'activated' using calcium and tissue thromboplastin

3.23 Disseminated intravascular coagulopathy (DIC) may be precipitated by

A Gram positive infection more commonly than Gram negative infection
B incompatible blood transfusion
C adenocarcinoma (mucin secreting)
D cardiac surgery
E placental abruption

3.24 When weaning an adult from a ventilator in ITU

A the PaO_2 must be greater than 11 kPa with an FiO_2 of 0.4 to have a reasonable chance of success
B the resting minute volume should be greater than 10 l/min
C SIMV stands for Spontaneous and Intermittent Mandatory Ventilation
D PEEP should not be used
E a tracheostomy makes weaning more difficult

3.25 Regarding double lumen tracheal tubes

A a Carlen tube is a right sided tube
B a Robertshaw tube has a carinal hook
C a White tube has a carinal hook and is a right sided tube
D a Bronchocath is available for right and left sides
E endobronchial blockers are inserted under direct vision

3.26 Carbon monoxide poisoning results in

A carbon monoxide inhibiting cellular respiration by binding to cytochromes
B a normal PaO_2
C a decreased SpO_2 detected by a pulse oximeter
D the possible need for hyperbaric oxygen
E carboxyhaemoglobin as carbon monoxide has an affinity for haemoglobin 150 times greater than oxygen

3.27 A severe burn may cause

A   large increases in plasma potassium following the administration of
    suxamethonium within a few minutes of the burn occurring
B   resistance to non-depolarising muscle relaxants
C   a peak rise in basal metabolic rate at 2 days
D   a rise in core temperature of 1-2°C
E   cyanide poisoning requiring treatment with amyl nitrate, thiosulphate
    or dicobalt edetate

3.28 The carcinoid syndrome may result in

A   diarrhoea
B   bronchospasm
C   pulmonary fibrosis
D   a raised urinary vanilyl mandelic acid
E   left sided cardiac valvular lesions

3.29 In the obese patient

A   morbid obesity may be defined as a body mass index (BMI) greater
    than 30
B   the intra-gastric pressure is raised but the residual gastric volume is
    normal
C   the functional residual capacity is reduced
D   the cardiac index is not elevated
E   opioids may be used on a normal mg/kg basis

3.30 Patient controlled analgesia

A   overcomes the large interpatient variation in opioid requirements
    following the same surgical procedure
B   allows a patient to maintain their plasma opioid levels around their
    individual minimum effective analgesic concentration (MEAC)
C   is improved if a background infusion is supplied
D   is not suitable for use in children under 12 years of age
E   may be provided by local anaesthetic agents via an epidural catheter

3.31 Gas flow

A becomes faster through a constriction
B is likely to be turbulent below a Reynolds number of 2000
C is dependent on the density of the gas when the flow is laminar
D through a rotameter at low flows is likely to be laminar as the gap around the bobbin represents an orifice
E is at a reduced pressure through a constriction, an effect used in Venturi oxygen masks

3.32 The characteristic facies of a patient with dystrophia myotonica include

A loss of the eyebrows
B ptosis
C a 'lateral smile'
D a malar erythematous rash
E a smooth forehead

3.33 Omphaloceles

A are more common than gastroschiasis
B are caused by intra-uterine occlusion of the omphalomesenteric artery
C are covered by a membrane
D are associated with other congenital malformations
E may necessitate parenteral nutrition in the neonate

3.34 Necrotizing enterocolitis

A has a similar nationwide incidence in special care baby units
B may be associated with multisystem failure
C can often be managed without surgical intervention
D occurs more commonly in premature low birth weight neonates
E has a low mortality

3.35 The following may raise intraocular pressure

A hypercarbia
B intravenous lignocaine
C β-blockers
D ecothiopate
E emesis

3.36 A retrobulbar block

A is performed using a standard 25 gauge needle
B requires 10 ml of 2% lignocaine
C may result in subarachnoid injection of local anaesthetic
D has, as a complication, retrobulbar haemorrhage which may necessitate cancellation of the procedure
E as a single injection results in an eye that is prepared for surgery

3.37 Limb tourniquets

A should be inflated to 100 mmHg above the systolic blood pressure when applied to the arm
B on the arm may be safely inflated for up to 2.5 hours
C result in a systemic metabolic alkalosis when deflated
D can lead to the development of ischaemic contractures
E are associated with cardiac arrest

3.38 When assessing the depth of anaesthesia

A Guedel's signs are of little use now that ether is rarely used
B the second stage of Guedel's signs is more likely to be seen following an inhalational than an intravenous induction
C a scoring system comprising heart rate, blood pressure, sweating, and lacrimation may be of use
D an individual's MAC requirement may be affected by premedicant agents
E it is known that MAC requirement is altered by the CSF sodium concentration

3.39 Adrenocortical deficiency

A may be a consequence of anticoagulant therapy
B may have an autoimmune aetiology
C often presents with hyperglycaemia
D is associated with a low intravascular volume
E is an indication for the perioperative administration of hydrocortisone

3.40 Regarding the brain death tests

A the pupillary responses test only the 2nd cranial nerves
B the corneal reflexes test the 5th and 7th cranial nerves
C a painful stimulus to the face tests the 5th and 7th cranial nerves
D the eyes remain in a fixed position within the orbit when the head is moved rapidly from side to side (doll's eye movement) in the presence of brain stem death
E the gag reflex tests the 9th, 10th, and 11th cranial nerves

3.41 During cardiopulmonary resuscitation of an adult

A resistant ventricular fibrillation may respond to defibrillation with one paddle on the chest and the other over the patient's back
B electromechanical dissociation (ECG complexes with no palpable output) may respond to bretylium tosylate
C 1 mg of adrenaline should be given every 5 minutes during a prolonged arrest
D bicarbonate may improve tissue oxygenation in the presence of hypoventilation
E bicarbonate administration represents a large sodium load

3.42 In patients with an atrial septal defect

A ostium primum is more common than ostium secondum
B the second heart sound is not split
C the murmur gets louder if pulmonary hypertension occurs
D ostium primum is associated with AV canal defects
E the defect is repaired via the left atrium

3.43 The incidence of perioperative deep venous thrombosis may be reduced by

A waiting for obese patients to lose weight before undertaking elective surgery
B epidural anaesthesia
C stopping smoking
D infusing aprotinin peroperatively
E using an inspired oxygen concentration greater than 0.5

3.44 **Children who arrive in hospital following a submersion incident (near-drowning)**

A have a low survival rate
B may present with a marked bradycardia and profound peripheral vasodilatation
C with fixed dilated pupils have a poor outcome
D have usually swallowed more water than they aspirated
E should not be ventilated with PEEP

3.45 **Thiopentone**

A is presented as a highly acidic solution
B is stored with 6% anhydrous sodium carbonate
C is stored in a nitrogen rich atmosphere
D results in reawakening as a consequence of rapid hepatic metabolism
E is mostly eliminated by being excreted unchanged by the kidney

3.46 **Myasthenia gravis may be associated with**

A rheumatoid arthritis
B pernicious anaemia
C thyrotoxicosis
D primary hyperaldosteronism
E frontal bossing

3.47 **Transcutaneous measurement of blood oxygen tension**

A measures the oxygen tension in arterial blood
B is likely to be inaccurate in high cardiac output states
C may result in cutaneous burns
D is a useful means of measuring blood oxygen tension in burned patients
E is sensitive to changes in temperature

3.48 **Regarding cerebral physiology**

    A a normal intracranial pressure (ICP) is 10-15 mmHg
    B central venous pressure at the jugular venous bulb is normally ~5 mmHg
    C autoregulation of cerebral blood flow occurs over the range of mean arterial pressure 30-120 mmHg
    D cerebral blood flow is primarily pressure dependent because the brain is relatively non-compliant
    E the prime determinant of cerebral blood flow is cerebral perfusion pressure

3.49 **The following are recognised risk factors for a significant cardiovascular perioperative event**

    A a fourth heart sound
    B a thoracic or abdominal surgical procedure
    C sinus arrhythmia
    D a previous CVA
    E an ejection fraction of 60%

3.50 **Blood pressure may be monitored using the following**

    A an arterial cannula whose internal lumen should taper at the end
    B a direct arterial system which is compliant and of small calibre
    C Korotkoff sounds
    D a blood pressure cuff that should have a width equal to 60% of the circumference of the limb
    E a Finapress

3.51 **The following are advantages of day surgery**

    A less time is needed for preoperative assessment
    B a decreased incidence of postoperative DVT
    C less disruption to a patient's life
    D less need to care for the patient postoperatively
    E lower medical costs

3.52 The following may cause perioperative seizures

A hypocarbia
B hypercalcaemia
C uraemia
D a low serum magnesium
E hyperpyrexia

3.53 In elderly patients

A there is a 50% loss of neuronal density by 80 years of age
B cerebral neurotransmitter levels are reduced
C cerebral O_2 consumption is unchanged
D the basal metabolic rate falls by 1% per year after the age of 45 years
E the glomerular filtration rate is approximately 60% of normal by 70 years of age

3.54 Regarding humidification

A absolute humidity is expressed as a percentage
B relative humidity is the actual amount of water vapour present in a volume of gas related to the maximum possible amount available at a specified temperature
C condensation occurs at the triple point
D humidification of dry inspired gases causes loss of body heat
E the partial pressure of O_2 decreases as inspired gas moves towards the alveoli

3.55 Humidification

A may be performed using a Boyle's bottle
B may be achieved by adding steam to inspired gases
C with a Venturi and baffle system results in the inhalation of large droplets
D may drown the patient
E decreases the risk of respiratory infection

3.56 In an acute attack of malignant hyperpyrexia

A the body temperature classically rises by 1°C per hour
B a raised body temperature is an early sign
C strabismus is a risk factor
D hypokalaemia is seen
E body metabolism is approximately five times normal

3.57 Malignant hyperpyrexia

A has an incidence of approximately 1 in 15 000
B is inherited as an autosomal recessive disorder
C results in muscle contractions precipitated by a high intracellular calcium
D may be precipitated by stress
E has its gene locus is on the long arm of chromosome 17

3.58 Hypertension

A has a prevalence of 1 in 7
B may result from alcohol abuse
C results in poor left ventricular relaxation
D may be seen in hypothyroidism
E is seen in Cushing's syndrome but not in Conn's syndrome

3.59 Hepatic blood flow

A may be decreased in association with hypocarbia
B is decreased with an increase in portal venous pressure
C is unlikely to be affected by intra-abdominal surgery
D falls during general and regional anaesthesia
E can be affected by metabolic and hormonal factors

3.60 Techniques which attenuate the hypertensive response to laryngoscopy include

A oral β-blockers with the premedicant
B intravenous lignocaine at induction
C a slow induction with ketamine to maintain cardiovascular stability
D intravenous morphine at induction
E spraying the vocal cords with lignocaine

3.61 Hypotensive anaesthesia results in

A a further fall in the FRC than that caused by anaesthesia alone
B failure of cerebral autoregulation if the mean arterial blood pressure (MABP) is <70 mmHg
C reduced glomerular filtration if the MABP is <60 mmHg
D loss of the cerebral vasoconstricting effect of hypocarbia if the MABP is <50 mmHg
E better maintenance of autoregulation if ganglion blockers are used rather than direct acting vasodilators

3.62 Downs syndrome

A is caused by meiotic non-dysjunction in 90% of cases
B is related to maternal age in 50% of cases
C rarely results in a difficult intubation
D may present with duodenal obstruction
E is associated with congenital heart disease in up to 20% of cases

3.63 Haemophilia A

A is a Y-linked recessive deficiency of Factor VIII
B results in a prolonged bleeding time
C is a contraindication to major surgery until Factor VIII levels are transfused to 25% of normal
D may be treated with DDAVP
E is an indication for epidural anaesthesia to control postoperative pain as intramuscular injections are contraindicated

3.64 During anaesthesia for laparoscopic sterilisation

A the FRC may fall by up to 20% with Trendelenburg positioning
B peritoneal traction is likely to result in tachycardia
C the volume of gas insufflated is usually 6 litres
D local anaesthesia alone may be adequate
E tracheal intubation if usually preferred

3.65 Laryngectomy patients

A may present a difficult intubation due to tissue scarring rather than the tumour mass
B often require preoperative lung function tests and arterial blood gases
C may require an initial tracheostomy under local anaesthesia
D should not receive an antisialagogue premedicant
E may require a simultaneous oesophagectomy

3.66 A classification system used to assess liver failure might usefully include

A the severity of ascites
B the bleeding time
C total plasma protein levels
D encephalopathy
E the presence of urinary urobilinogen

3.67 Systemic inflammatory response syndrome (SIRS)

A can occur without infection
B uses a white cell count of $<4 \times 10^9$ cm^{-3} as one of its possible diagnostic criteria
C will develop into multiple organ dysfunction syndrome in 70% of cases
D can be diagnosed with a heart rate of 70 beats per minute
E may be precipitated by Gram negative endotoxins which are lipopolysaccarides

3.68 Brain death tests

A must be performed simultaneously by two doctors
B must be performed by at least one doctor of consultant grade
C must always be performed twice with at least 2 hours between tests
D may be performed by a doctor who graduated 5 years previously
E should not be performed until 6 hours have elapsed since the event that caused suspected brain death

3.69 With regard to patients who have been burned

A prognosis depends on age and chronic health status
B one leg represents 9% of the body surface area
C a superficial partial thickness burn will heal in approximately 10 days if no infection occurs
D a full thickness burn heals by wound contraction
E the plasma oncotic pressure falls following a major burn

3.70 In the carcinoid syndrome

A treatment may include ketanserin
B regional anaesthesia may result in bradykinin release
C sympathomimetics should be used to treat perioperative hypotension
D direct arterial blood pressure monitoring is usually indicated
E metastases are normally found in the liver once the syndrome has developed

3.71 During labour

A uterine afferents enter the spinal cord from T_{10} to S_1
B TENS uses a frequency of 500Hz
C entonox provides adequate relief for 60% of mothers
D midwives may give pethidine without a doctor's prescription
E the effects on the fetus of maternal intramuscular pethidine will have
   worn off by 3 hours

**3.72 The following may cause an adult respiratory distress syndrome
(ARDS)**

A smoke inhalation
B oxygen toxicity
C pancreatitis
D cardiopulmonary bypass
E asthma

3.73 The following occur commonly in pre-eclampsia

A double vision
B upper abdominal pain
C constipation
D dyspnoea
E hyporeflexia

3.74 Pre-eclampsia

A is a contraindication to vaginal delivery
B is an indication for epidural analgesia provided that the bleeding time
   is normal
C may be associated with a difficult intubation
D may be treated with magnesium sulphate which results in the need for
   increased doses of neuromuscular blockers
E is an indication for insertion of a subclavian line

3.75 Cardiopulmonary bypass

A may be performed using the femoral vessels
B requires a 'priming' volume of approximately 2 litres of blood
C usually results in a fall in the mean arterial blood pressure to 40 mmHg
   as bypass commences
D is inefficient at CO_2 removal
E requires 6 mg/kg of heparin to be given

3.76 Myocardial oxygen delivery is dependent upon

A heart rate
B systolic blood pressure
C left ventricular end systolic pressure
D left ventricular end diastolic volume
E haemoglobin concentration

3.77 Soda lime

A contains 20% sodium hydroxide
B requires moisture for its chemical reactions to occur
C contains 1% potassium hydroxide
D produces heat when absorbing CO_2
E contains 75% calcium hydroxide

3.78 Anaemia in renal failure

A is usually hypochromic and hypocytic
B may be associated with a prolonged bleeding time
C is rarely treated with erythropoietin as it reduces the likelihood of a successful transplant in the future
D is usually caused by chronic blood loss
E may be corrected whilst being haemodialysed

3.79 In a patient being anaesthetised for renal transplantation

A suxamethonium should not be used
B Hartmann's solution should initially be used to replace fluid loss
C neuromuscular blockade monitoring should always be used
D CVP and arterial lines are always necessary
E hypotension is treated with α-adrenergic agonists in preference to fluids

3.80 The following are identified by Goldmann as risk factors for a peroperative myocardial event

A a third heart sound
B age >55
C intra-peritoneal surgery
D a myocardial infarction within 2 years
E a raised CVP

3.81 APACHE III scoring

A further simplifies APACHE II scoring by using less physiological variables

B includes function and co-morbidity scoring in the chronic health evaluation

C increases the number of diagnostic categories available to 230

D allows outcome to be predicted for ITU patients as a group

E assesses use of resources

3.82 Ascites

A classically causes decreased bowel sounds in the flanks

B is treated with a salt losing diuretic

C may require a peritoneovenous shunt

D may be caused by cardiac failure

E has no important anaesthetic implications

3.83 Sedation in the intensive care unit

A using morphine may result in accumulation of its metabolite morphine-6-glucuronidine

B for patients with renal failure is best achieved using pethidine

C commonly leads to withdrawal symptoms

D is very effectively produced using diazepam

E may occasionally necessitate thiopentone infusion

3.84 Preoperative

A investigation should include a haemoglobin in all patients over 60 years of age

B starvation by omitting food for 6 hours in all patients is mandatory

C tests are best if sensitivity is greater than specificity

D spirometry has a normal FEV_1/FVC ratio of 60%

E a chest X-ray should be obtained in patients over 70

3.85 Epidural analgesia during labour

A may be administered using a patient controlled analgesic device

B results in a higher operative delivery rate if epidural opioids are used

C may cause bradycardia if the block extends to T_6

D will cause a headache in 95% of patients if a dural tap is performed with a 16G Tuohy needle

E results in a dural puncture in approximately 4% of women

3.86 **In pregnant patients**

    A motilin secretion is decreased
    B gastric emptying is unaffected
    C gastrin levels are unchanged
    D precautions against the risk of aspiration should be taken from the 18th week
    E gastric emptying is affected by labour

3.87 **Regional anaesthesia for the obese patient**

    A should be used whenever possible
    B will require the normal mg/kg drug doses
    C avoids the necessity to give postoperative oxygen
    D is associated with blocks of unpredictable height and onset
    E may be used even if a history of sleep apnoea is obtained

3.88 **A pregnant woman receiving an anaesthetic at 24 weeks gestation**

    A may receive either atropine or glycopyrrolate as neither crosses the placenta
    B should be hyperventilated to a greater extent than her physiological hyperventilation
    C does not require tocographic monitoring as it is rarely possible at this stage of gestation
    D does not need to be placed in a left lateral tilt position whilst supine
    E should if possible have a regional rather than a general anaesthetic

3.89 **Regarding muscle relaxants**

    A phase II block may occur with as little as 3 mg/kg of suxamethonium
    B post-tetanic facilitation does not occur with a phase II block
    C a dibucaine number of 50 suggests that the patient is homozygous for abnormal cholinesterase genes
    D ten genotypes for cholinesterase may be found
    E patients with poliomyelitis show a normal duration of action with non-depolarising muscle relaxants

3.90 Acute diabetic ketoacidosis

A may necessitate surgery before metabolic control can be obtained
B is treated with 5% glucose once the blood sugar is 10 mmol/l
C is associated with a total body excess of potassium
D usually requires at least 1 litre of 0.9% saline to be given in the first hour after presentation
E may, in severe cases, necessitate intubation and ventilation at 70-100 ml/kg/min at least for the first 24 hours

PRACTICE PAPER FOUR

Allow 3 hours for the completion of all 90 questions
Answers are on page 117

4.1 **In a patient with well controlled epilepsy who requires a general anaesthetic**

A anticonvulsants should be omitted only on the day of operation
B metoclopramide is contraindicated
C methohexitone should not be used
D ketamine is contraindicated
E curare may cause seizure activity

4.2 **Anaemia may be caused by**

A glucose-6-phosphate dehydrogenase deficiency
B uraemia
C prosthetic heart valves
D splenectomy
E thyroid hormone deficiency

4.3 **When assessing patients with asthma prior to anaesthesia**

A a chest X-ray usually provides valuable information
B disease severity is best assessed by measuring pulmonary gas transfer
C ECG changes are usually only present in severe cases
D pulmonary function tests may show considerable variation at different times of day
E an elevated $PaCO_2$ may be normal in the majority of asthmatics

4.4 **Nitrous oxide**

A is stored as a gas at room temperature
B supports combustion
C has no colour and is non-irritant to the respiratory tract
D cannot be detected using infra-red gas analysers
E is a sympathomimetic and increases systemic vascular resistance

4.5 Myasthenia gravis

A is a diagnosis confirmed by the finding of a high titre of anti-acetyl-choline receptor antibodies

B produces fade and post-tetanic facilitation on testing with a nerve stimulator

C may present as a myasthenic crisis if the patient takes an excessive dose of anticholinesterase

D is usually associated with a normal response to depolarising muscle relaxants

E is associated with a thymoma in more than 50% of sufferers

4.6 A blood transfusion

A may depress immune function

B cannot transmit parasitic infections

C may result in non-haemolytic reactions

D leads to some form of reaction in 3-5% of patients

E can cause hand, foot and mouth disease in the immunocompromised patient by transmission of the Epstein-Barr virus

4.7 Mitral regurgitation

A may be associated with mitral stenosis

B results in concentric hypertrophy of the left ventricle

C causes an ejection systolic murmur radiating to the axilla

D may result in pulmonary hypertension and right ventricular failure

E is a cause of a third heart sound

4.8 In a patient with a chronic cervical transection

A a rapid sequence induction with muscle relaxation provided by a non-depolarising agent, or an awake intubation should always be performed if a general anaesthetic is given

B autonomic hyperreflexia may be exacerbated by spinal anaesthesia

C spinal reflexes often necessitate the use of muscle relaxants if a general anaesthetic is given

D sedative premedication should be given

E antisialagogue agents are contraindicated

4.9 In the head injured patient with elevated intracranial pressure, cerebral perfusion may be safely increased by

A the use of PEEP
B ventilating the patient to a state of hypercarbia
C drainage of CSF
D the intravenous administration of mannitol
E the administration of a barbiturate such as thiopentone

4.10 Preoperative temporary cardiac pacing is required in the following

A Mobitz type II second degree heart block
B bifasicular heart block that is asymptomatic
C sinus node disease
D Mobitz type I second degree heart block
E 1st degree heart block

4.11 In dystrophia myotonica, myotonia may be precipitated by

A isoflurane
B exercise
C hypokalaemia
D neostigmine
E suxamethonium

4.12 In comparison with adults, infants have

A a low pulse rate and low blood pressure
B a larynx which is narrowest at the level of the thyroid cartilage
C a high oxygen consumption on a weight basis
D a greater resistance to the respiratory depressant effects of opioids
E an increased extracellular fluid volume

4.13 In the elderly patient

A the compliance of the vascular trees increases with increasing age
B baroreceptor sensitivity is unchanged
C sympathetic tone is reduced
D stroke volume is reduced
E total body water is increased

4.14 Pyloric stenosis

  A is the commonest neonatal problem presenting for surgery
  B has an incidence of 1:600
  C has an equal sex incidence
  D usually presents at the age of one month
  E is caused by an intrauterine viral infection

4.15 An active gas scavenging system

  A collects waste gas from the 22 mm male conical connector on the
     breathing system or ventilator
  B does not require a positive pressure relief valve as the system runs with
     negative pressure
  C usually incorporates an air brake
  D can be powered using a venturi system
  E should be able to tolerate peak gas flows of 130 l/min

4.16 Spinal anaesthesia

  A improves long term postoperative mortality in fixation of a fractured
     neck of femur when compared with general anaesthesia
  B results in a constricted small bowel
  C is contraindicated if a pericardial effusion is present
  D is absolutely contraindicated in multiple sclerosis
  E acts primarily on nerve roots rather than the spinal cord

4.17 The diving reflex

  A is not seen in children
  B is associated with a marked tachycardia
  C is associated with intense peripheral vasoconstriction
  D involves the trigeminal nerves in its afferent pathway
  E involves the vagus nerves in its efferent pathway

4.18 When anaesthetising patients with a phaeochromocytoma

  A premedication with atropine should be avoided
  B intravenous fluid administration should be restricted
  C halothane is the volatile agent of choice as it causes the least
     haemodynamic instability
  D hypoglycaemia may be encountered in the postoperative period
  E a noradrenaline infusion may be required in the postoperative period

4.19 During general anaesthesia

A the ventilatory response to CO_2 is depressed to a greater extent than the response to hypoxia

B diaphragmatic function is preserved to a greater extent than that of the chest wall muscles

C atelectasis is more likely to occur if N_2O is added to the inspired gas

D the use of PEEP will prevent the occurrence of dependent atelectasis

E enflurane depresses respiration more than halothane

4.20 Permanent cardiac pacemakers

A are classified using a code in which the first letter refers to the cardiac chamber that is sensed

B classified as VOO are in a fixed pacing mode

C may produce cannon waves in the jugular venous pulse

D should be removed as an emergency procedure if the patient requires urgent d.c. cardioversion

E are an indication for prophylactic peroperative antibiotic cover

4.21 The liver

A receives 15% of the cardiac output

B blood flow is not decreased during regional anaesthesia

C metabolizes approximately 10% of inspired halothane

D enzymes may be induced by barbiturates

E receives 70% of its blood from the portal vein

4.22 In transposition of the great arteries

A an 'egg shaped' heart is seen on the chest X-ray

B two independent parallel circulation's occur

C atrial balloon septoplasty is performed after six months of age

D is associated with intrauterine viral infection

E correction requires the switching of the coronary arteries as well as the great vessels

4.23 Within SI units of measurement

A temperature is measured in degrees Centigrade

B the Newton is a unit of energy

C the amount of a substance is measured in moles

D one Pascal equals 1 Newton acting over 1 square metre

E there are five basic units with others being derived from them

4.24 The following drugs are usually discontinued prior to anaesthesia and major surgery

A sulphonylureas
B benzodiazepines
C the combined oral contraceptive pill
D coumarins
E Angiotensin converting enzyme (ACE) inhibitors

4.25 Using patient controlled analgesia

A patients will, if possible, take enough opioid to entirely remove their pain
B respiratory depression may occur
C some degree of sedation is common
D drug addiction is more likely than using an intramuscular regimen
E loading doses are not necessary as the patient is able to take enough opioid to rapidly remove pain

4.26 Congenital tracheoesophageal fistulae

A are rarely associated with other congenital abnormalities
B may be suspected in utero following a finding of oligohydramnios
C should, if possible, be repaired with in 2 days of diagnosis
D are most safely isolated following intubation after an intravenous induction of anaesthesia
E usually require a chest drain to be sited preoperatively

4.27 Congenital diaphragmatic herniae

A are more common in males than females
B are found on the left side in 80% of cases
C compress the otherwise normal lung
D are associated with pulmonary hypertension
E are an indication for avoiding nitrous oxide during an anaesthetic

4.28 Nitric oxide

A is also known as endothelial derived relaxing factor
B is found in striated muscle
C has a half life of 30 seconds
D acts by decreasing intracellular cyclic guanosine monophosphate
E is produced from L-arginine by nitric oxide synthase

4.29 **The following agents lower intraocular pressure**

A nitrous oxide
B propofol
C curare
D acetazolamide
E ketamine

4.30 **When cement is used during a total hip replacement**

A hypotension is reduced if a cement gun is employed
B preloading with fluid should be routinely performed prior to cementing
C hypotension may be the result of cement entering the circulation
D allergy to the cement is relatively common
E it may have antibiotics added to it

4.31 **Scoliosis**

A is most commonly idiopathic in aetiology
B is associated with pulmonary hypertension
C surgery is a contraindication to a hypotensive anaesthetic technique as the cardiovascular system may be compromised by the scoliosis
D corrective surgery may necessitate the use of a double lumen tracheal tube
E surgery may require the patient to be wakened during the operative procedure

4.32 **Acute epiglottitis**

A is usually caused by infection with respiratory syncitial virus (RSV)
B has a peak incidence in children below the age of 2 years
C requires a lateral neck X-ray for the diagnosis to be confirmed
D causes the child to drool saliva and is thus an indication for premedication with atropine
E is best managed by intubation under deep halothane anaesthesia if control of the airway is required

4.33 Adverse drug reactions during anaesthesia

A are usually predictable and a consequence of the known pharmacological actions of the agent
B may occur in otherwise healthy individuals
C may be related to an immune response on behalf of the patient
D may be life-threatening
E occur more frequently in those patients known to be atopic

4.34 Regarding investigation of the cardiovascular system

A ECG stress testing with ST segment depression of 0.5 mV is an indication for further investigation
B 70% of patients with radiological cardiomegaly have an ejection fraction < 50%
C two-dimensional echocardiography is better than M mode for examination of valve structure
D akinetic areas of ventricular wall pose more risk during anaesthesia than hypokinetic areas
E a MUGA scan is an invasive technique with similar risks to angiography

4.35 While investigating a patient for malignant hyperpyrexia

A a normal creatinine phosphokinase excludes the diagnosis
B a muscle biopsy is usually performed under local anaesthesia
C biopsied muscle from a patient who is MH susceptible develops a contraction of 2 g force when exposed to 2% halothane or 2 mmol/l of caffeine
D creatinine phosphokinase levels may be used as an initial test for screening family members
E the effect of dantrolene on ionised plasma calcium levels may be helpful

4.36 When using Mallampati's airway assessment

A the mouth should be examined from behind the head (intubating position)
B a tongue depressor is used to permit greater assessment of the pharynx
C when only the soft palate, faucial pillars, and uvula are seen the patient is graded as Class 2
D the patient can only be graded accurately after direct laryngoscopy
E a lateral head/neck X-ray will confirm the assessment

4.37 Regarding enteral nutrition

A in the presence of a normal colon, enteral nutrition is possible with as little as 25 cm of small bowel
B the ideal enteral feed for a non-catabolic adult should provide around 2000 kcal per day
C the ideal enteral feed for a non-catabolic adult should provide around 9 g of protein per day
D lactase is an important constituent of enteral feeds in post-surgical patients
E carbohydrates in enteral feeds are usually supplied as maltodextrins

4.38 The following are associated with diabetes mellitus

A atlanto-axial disease in type I diabetes
B phaeochromocytoma
C pulmonary fibrosis
D cardiomyopathy
E hyperthyroidism

4.39 Regarding oxygen transport

A oxygen content is the volume of oxygen present and is measured in ml
B oxygen flux is the oxygen delivered to the tissues per minute
C available oxygen is the oxygen content divided by the cardiac output
D the volume of dissolved oxygen is equal to 0.00225 ml x PaO_2 (measured in kPa)
E a haemoglobin of approximately 14 g/dl provides optimal tissue oxygen delivery

4.40 The following statements about ventilators are correct

A a pressure generator is unaffected by a change in lung compliance
B the pressure produced by a flow generator is constant
C cycling may be determined by time, pressure, volume or flow
D a Penlon Nuffield 200 requires an electrical supply
E a cuirass generates a negative pressure

4.41 Marfan's syndrome

A is an inherited connective tissue disorder
B may cause arachnoiditis
C may be associated with downward dislocation of the ocular lens
D represents no particular anaesthetic difficulties apart from the increased risk of pneumothorax
E can result in a twisted sternum and muscle hypotonia

4.42 Pneumoperitoneum during laparoscopy for gynaecological surgery

A usually necessitates intra-abdominal pressures of 40 cmH$_2$O
B may cause a pneumothorax
C may result in a pneumopericardium
D may be produced using nitrogen
E is a possible cause of perioperative acidosis

4.43 Regarding the instrumental monitoring of the depth of anaesthesia

A cortical evoked potentials are more susceptible to depression by anaesthesia than brain stem evoked potentials
B lower oesophageal contractility is a useful technique provided that the patient has not been given muscle relaxants
C the electroencephalogram (EEG) is a sensitive measure of the depth of anaesthesia
D the isolated forearm technique involves applying a tourniquet above the systolic blood pressure to the arm before muscle relaxants are given
E skin conductance is a quantification of sweat gland activity and may be correlated to the depth of anaesthesia

4.44 Percutaneous dilational tracheostomy

A was first described by Ciaglia
B should be performed in the operating theatre
C requires two physicians, at least one of which should be an anaesthetist
D should be sited immediately below the cricoid cartilage
E is a Seldinger technique

4.45 Carbon dioxide

A   absorbs infra-red light
B   in blood is measured directly by the CO_2 electrode of a blood gas analyser
C   measurement in expired gases may be inaccurate in the presence of nitrous oxide
D   measurement in expired gases may be inaccurate in the presence of nitric oxide
E   produces narcosis when its concentration in inspired gases is greater than 10%

4.46 In patients with an inhalational burn

A   throbbing headache, nausea, and vomiting may suggest carbon monoxide poisoning
B   except following inhalation of steam, mucosal injury is usually confined to the supra-glottic airway
C   pulse oximetry is essential in those with significant levels of carboxyhaemoglobin as conventional blood gas analysis is inaccurate under such conditions
D   amyl nitrate may be given if there is evidence of cyanide poisoning
E   hyperbaric oxygen therapy is a recognised treatment in cases of severe cyanide poisoning

4.47 Risk factors for the development of a perioperative deep venous thrombosis include

A   antithrombin III deficiency
B   nephrotic syndrome
C   varicose veins
D   Lupus disease
E   hypotensive anaesthesia

4.48 The following may be considered desirable properties of the 'ideal' inhalational anaesthetic agent

A   a high potency
B   a high blood gas solubility
C   a high biotransformation
D   a boiling point between 0-10°C
E   a low MAC

4.49　Halothane

A　is chemically unstable
B　has a MAC value of 0.87 in neonates
C　has a boiling point of 50°C
D　is 2% metabolised by the liver
E　is stored with 1% thymol

4.50　The following may be beneficial following an accidental intra-arterial injection of thiopentone

A　cooling the limb
B　stellate ganglion block
C　noradrenaline infusion
D　administration of papaverine
E　administration of phenoxybenzamine

4.51　The following are predictive of difficulty with intubation

A　Singh-Vaughan-Williams class 3
B　a ratio of mandibular length:posterior depth of >3.6 on a radiograph
C　a thyromental distance of >6.5 cm
D　a reduced distance between the spinous process of C_1 and the occiput
E　a reduced distance from the tip of the most anterior incisor to the bottom of the mandible

4.52　During cardiopulmonary resuscitation of an adult

A　a precordial thump should be given to all patients who require advanced life support
B　a precordial thump may be of benefit in pulseless ventricular tachycardia and torsade de pointes
C　ventricular fibrillation requires defibrillation commencing at 50 J
D　adrenaline should be the first drug to be given in the case of asystole
E　intracardiac injection represents the best route of administration of adrenaline in the case of asystole

4.53 Light emitting from a laser source

A consists of two parallel wavelengths when the source is carbon dioxide
B is in the red region of the visible spectrum when the source is carbon dioxide
C has a wavelength of ~500 nm when the source is argon
D may be transmitted around corners using fibreoptics
E may penetrate mucous membranes up to a depth of 1 cm when the source is carbon dioxide

4.54 Signs that a patient with raised intracranial pressure is decompensating include

A hypertension
B photophobia
C nausea and vomiting
D oliguria
E neck stiffness

4.55 With regard to local anaesthesia of the upper airway

A Krause's method is a technique for performing a glossopharyngeal nerve block
B a maxillary nerve block may be performed via the sphenopalatine canal
C the superior laryngeal nerve may be blocked at the greater cornu of the hyoid bone
D the superior laryngeal nerve may be blocked via the mucosa of the piriform fossa
E the mucosa supplied by the superior laryngeal nerve may be anaesthetised by injecting local anaesthetic through the cricothyroid membrane

4.56 A fuel cell used to measure the partial pressure of oxygen in a gas mixture

A relies on the fact that oxygen is paramagnetic
B employs a gold cathode
C requires a voltage of 0.6 V to be applied between its electrodes
D consumes electrons at its anode as oxygen reacts with them
E is sensitive to changes in temperature

4.57 Errors in pulse oximetry may arise in the presence of

A nail varnish
B methylene blue
C tricuspid incompetence
D methaemoglobin
E carboxyhaemoglobin

4.58 Regarding the prevention of cross contamination between patients

A 10% sodium hypochlorite has only minimal antiviral activity
B glutaraldehyde may leave a toxic residue
C boiling for 5 minutes will effectively sterilize items
D chlorhexidine 0.05% is the agent of choice for cleaning following a
   spillage of HIV positive blood
E pasteurization is a method of decontamination

4.59 Body temperature

A demonstrates a circadian rhythm with the peak at 1200 hours
B is maintained with heat produced by muscle movement alone
C is controlled via the hypothalamus
D can be measured in degrees centigrade with absolute zero being 0°C
E may be monitored via a pulmonary artery catheter

4.60 With regard to ABO blood groups

A group O is found in 38% of the population
B group AB patients have no plasma antibodies of the ABO system
C group AB is found in 15% of the population
D group O patients are universal donors having both anti-A and anti-B
   plasma antibodies
E 75% of patients are secretors for the ABO system with evidence of
   their blood group being seen in urine, saliva, or sweat

4.61 Hypothermia results in

A a right shift of the oxygen dissociation curve
B pupils that are fixed and dilated below 28°C
C hypoglycaemia
D decreased hypoxic pulmonary vasoconstriction
E delta waves in the ECG

4.62 Suction

A for peroperative surgical use should provide high negative pressures with a low displacement

B for postoperative wound drainage is usually of low pressure and displacement

C needs to generate a maximally negative pressure of -200 mmHg to be appropriate for anaesthetic usage

D can be generated using a venturi system

E for multiple piped outlets works off a large central reservoir tank

4.63 During the treatment of SIRS

A infection should only be treated when antibiotic sensitivity is known

B inverse I:E ratios increase the incidence of barotrauma

C permissive hypercapnia should not be used

D glutamine is given to protect renal function

E lactic acidaemia correlates with poor outcome

4.64 An antisialagogue premedicant

A is contraindicated in patients for oral surgery

B should not be given if ketamine is to be used

C may increase the risk of inspissation of bronchial secretions

D has no unpleasant side effects

E should always be used in neonates

4.65 Multiple sclerosis

A is best diagnosed by CSF examination

B is more common in women

C most commonly presents in patients over 40 years of age

D often presents with transient neurological deficits

E is more common in tropical countries

4.66 Lower motor neurone lesions occur in the following

A spinal cord injury

B motor neurone disease

C Cushing's syndrome

D multiple sclerosis

E myasthenia gravis

4.67 **Suxamethonium should be avoided in**

A patients with hypokalaemia
B multiple sclerosis
C motor neurone disease
D the immediate management of a high spinal cord injury
E Conn's syndrome

4.68 **An acute attack of porphyria**

A may present with psychosis
B rarely involves the nervous system
C can cause abdominal pain
D includes a severe exacerbation of skin manifestations
E may be precipitated by stress

4.69 **Carotid artery surgery**

A leaves the contralateral hemisphere dependent on perfusion from the Circle of Willis when the carotid artery is clamped
B carotid stump pressures (after cross clamping) of <70 mmHg indicate the need for a temporary shunt
C may be performed under local anaesthesia
D is performed without heparinization as this may increase the risk of a CVA
E is associated with reduced autonomic stimulation when local anaesthetic is infiltrated around the carotid body

4.70 **The vomiting centre**

A lies just outside the blood-brain barrier
B receives afferent nerve fibres from the cerebrum
C has noradrenaline as its predominant neurotransmitter
D is closely associated with the chemoreceptor trigger zone lying in the posterior wall of the fourth ventricle
E is found within the reticular formation in the medulla

4.71 The following are particular complications of transurethral resection of the prostate (TURP)

    A burns
    B fibrinolysis
    C iso-osmolar volume overload
    D hypothermia
    E postoperative shoulder tip pain

4.72 Aortic stenosis

    A resulting from calcification usually occurs on a tricuspid valve
    B commonly presents with syncope
    C results in a waterhammer pulse
    D does not affect ventricular compliance
    E leads to hypertrophic dilation of the left ventricle

4.73 Universal precautions

    A means that all patients are assumed to be 'infective'
    B means that gloves should be warn for any patient contact
    C should include the wearing of a protective gown if infective fluids may be splashed
    D are applied to hepatitis B positive patients
    E includes the use of goggles and masks

4.74 Air embolism

    A is more likely if the CVP is low
    B may occur during an arthrogram
    C is more serious if the rate of air entrainment is slow and gradual rather than rapid
    D occurs in up to 25% of sitting neurosurgical cases
    E may occur during suction termination of pregnancy

4.75 When blood is stored

    A adenosine triphosphate (ATP) levels fall
    B osmotic fragility decreases
    C potassium will rise to 20 mmol/l by 21 days
    D pH may fall below 7.0
    E clotting is impaired to a clinically significant degree within 24 hours of donation

4.76 Regarding haematological tests

A the bleeding time measures the ability of blood to clot
B platelet function may be assessed with adenosine diphosphate (ADP), collagen or thrombin
C a normal fibrinogen level is >300 mg/100 ml
D fibrin degradation products are tested for using serial dilution techniques
E the thrombin time tests the final common pathway and has a normal result of 9-15 seconds

4.77 The following are diagnostic criteria for disseminated intravascular coagulopathy

A a fibrinogen level <50 mg/100 ml
B a platelet count <150 000/ml^3
C a prothrombin time >25 seconds
D the presence of fibrin degradation products
E a normal thrombin time

4.78 For a diagnosis of brain death to be made

A the PaCO$_2$ must be markedly elevated
B hyponatraemia must be corrected
C the formal brain death tests may be performed if the pupils are fixed and dilated while the patient is breathing with a tracheal tube in situ
D the cause of irreversible brain damage should be known
E hypotension must be corrected

4.79 In patients with a ventricular septal defect

A a dacron patch repair can be performed without cardiopulmonary bypass
B Eisenmenger's syndrome occurs if the shunt reverses
C the defect will close spontaneously in nearly all cases if the lesion is small
D the loudness of the murmur is proportional to the size of the defect
E the chest X-ray will show small pulmonary arteries

4.80 Early intubation following a burn is indicated if

A there are full thickness burns of the lips or nose
B there are extensive burns to the chest
C severe cyanide poisoning is diagnosed
D 20% of the haemoglobin is converted to carboxyhaemoglobin
E a steam burn has occurred as this may extend into the bronchial tree

4.81 In patients with cardiovascular disease

A up to 25% of myocardial infarctions are asymptomatic
B most patients with untreated hypertension develop symptoms
C anaesthesia and surgery within 6 months of a myocardial infarction is typically associated with a reinfarction rate of 6.5%
D invasive monitoring and close control of haemodynamic variables decreases the reinfarction rate during anaesthesia following a recent myocardial infarction
E a physician's clinical findings correlate well with measured haemodynamic variables

4.82 Nitrous oxide

A has a MAC value of 95%
B cylinders have a pressure gauge which gives useful information about the contents of the cylinder only when the valve is closed
C cannot be measured by mass spectrometry as it consists of more than one type of atom
D may be measured by an infra-red analyser because it consists of more than one type of atom
E requires the cylinder tare weight to be known before an estimate of the contents of a cylinder may be made

4.83 Sevoflurane

A is a halogenated hydrocarbon
B is a molecule halogenated with only fluoride ions
C may prove to be especially useful for the inhalational induction of anaesthesia
D is flammable in clinically useful concentrations
E requires a special pressurised vaporiser

4.84 Propofol

A is a suitable induction agent for patients with porphyria
B is presented as a hypotonic solution
C is a suitable induction agent for patients who are susceptible to malignant hyperthermia
D undergoes conjugation in the liver
E is primarily excreted in bile

4.85 The following are appropriate in the immediate management of an anaphylactoid/anaphylactic reaction during anaesthesia

A high dose intravenous frusemide
B cessation of all intravenous infusions
C increasing the concentration of inspired anaesthetic vapour to deepen anaesthesia
D intramuscular adrenaline (50-100 µg)
E intravenous bicarbonate

4.86 Aldosterone

A is the principal glucocorticoid produced by the adrenal gland
B is secreted by the zona fasiculata
C causes sodium loss at the kidney
D causes hydrogen loss at the kidney
E is released following the conversion of renin to angiotensin

4.87 When considering postoperative analgesia

A the equipotent oral dose of morphine is 200-300% of the parenteral dose
B accidental swallowing of sublingual buprenorphine is potentially dangerous as there is a much enhanced bioavailability
C intercostal cryoanalgesia may be performed during thoracotomy but will not provide pain relief in the area served by the anterior primary rami of the intercostal nerve
D trichloroethylene is an analgesic volatile agent with a high blood gas solubility
E transcutaneous nerve stimulation (TENS) has not been shown to reduce the analgesic requirement in postoperative surgical patients

4.88 The catabolic phase associated with the stress response to surgery

A may commence preoperatively
B may last for up to 5 days
C results in sodium loss
D has no effect on free fatty acids
E results in decreased blood flow to skin and fatty tissues

4.89 Lung resection

A is contraindicated if the FEV_1 is <0.8 l/min
B results in secretion retention if the FEV_1 is <1.5 l/min
C is associated with the loss of 20% of lung function per lobe
D is an indication for preoperative pulmonary artery catheterisation to assess the probable respiratory effects of the proposed surgery
E of a lobe has a perioperative mortality of 2-3%

4.90 A bronchopleural fistula

A is likely to occur in up to 10% of patients following pneumonectomy
B is rarely associated with an empyema
C may present with the sudden onset of a productive cough
D is an absolute indication for a preoperative chest drain
E is an indication for a gaseous induction

ANSWERS TO PAPER ONE

The correct stems appear in bold
References refer to page numbers in *Key Topics in Anaesthesia* second edition

1.1 **A C D E** p.259
B   hypochloraemic alkalosis

1.2 **C E** p.52
A   the heart is stopped in diastole
B   20 mmol/l
D   it is ice cold

1.3 **A B D** p.285
C   elimination from the CSF is by vascular uptake

1.4 **B C D E** p.287
A   ephedrine is an alpha and beta adrenoreceptor agonist, methoxamine is
a purely alpha

1.5 **B C D** p.268
A   halogenated volatile agents are absorbed by activated charcoal, but not
nitrous oxide
B   calcium hydroxide 90%, sodium hydroxide 5%, potassium hydroxide
1%, silicates and an indicator

1.6 **C** p.93
A   the osmolality is ~1000 mOsm/kg
B   each gram of nitrogen is matched by 100-125 kcal of energy
E   there is no place for hyperalimentation

1.7 **C D E** p.213
A   tracheal tube size (mm) after 1 year = (age x 0.25) + 4.0
B   tracheal tube length (cm) after 1 year = (age x 0.5) + 12

1.8 **A B D** p.223

1.9 **A B C D** p.132

1.10 **A B D** p.223
C   the patient's blood pressure should be adequately controlled and the
vascular compartment rehydrated preoperatively over several days
E   a patient with a phaeochromocytoma is usually hypovolaemic at
presentation

1.11   **D** p.4
        A   mast cell degranulation may result from a direct pharmacological
             effect
        B   such a reaction is more likely to be anaphylactoid
        C   IgE
        E   testing should only be performed with full resuscitation facilities

1.12   **A** p.1
        B   fluid overload is more likely
        C   hypokalaemia
        D   hyperglycaemia

1.13   **B C D** p.294
        A   up to five times the preoperative level
        E   growth hormone is released by the pituitary

1.14   **B C** p.304
        A   low V:Q ratio
        D   the FEV_1:FVC ratio is reduced

1.15   **A C D E** p.49
        B   a raised intracranial pressure causes arrhythmias

1.16   **A D E** p.308
        B, C   these are relative indications and are a surgical luxury
        A, D, E   in these examples a double lumen tube will help control
                   airway soiling and air leak

1.17   **B** p.37
        A   neither direct nor consensual reactions are seen
        C   the corneal reflex tests the 5th and 7th nerves
        D   no nystagmus is seen if brain death is diagnosed
        E   no eye movement is seen, the eyes remain in a fixed position within
             the orbit if brain death is diagnosed

1.18   **A E** p.100
        B   at low flows a tubular orifice with laminar flow occurs
        C   it is present to make it easier to see that the bobbin is spinning
        D   it protects the vaporisers and flowmeters

1.19 **B** p.213

   A   it has no valve

   C   three times the minute ventilation should be used

   D   it does not

   E   providing the reservoir of the 'T' piece is of a large enough capacity and the fresh gas flow is high enough, there is no upper weight limit restricting its use

1.20 **C D** p.294

   B   the effect does not last into the postoperative period

   E   the obtunding effect wears off when the epidural does

1.21 **A C D** p.169

   E   survival to the sixth decade is usual

1.22 **A D** p.225

   B   number of atoms in 12 g of carbon

   C   it occupies 22.4 litres at standard temperature and pressure

   E   after 2 time constants 86.5% of the original value remains

1.23 **C** p.197

   A   surgery should, if possible, be delayed until the stomach is empty and the patient is resuscitated from any other injuries

   B   the rise in IOP following suxamethonium is short lived

   D   even then the stomach may not have emptied, especially if the patient is in pain from other injuries

1.24 **A C D E** p.203

   A   but it does support combustion

   B   -119°C

1.25 **B C E** pp.47, 78, 169, 266, 167

1.26 **C D E** p.174

   A   it is not associated with other abnormalities

1.27 **A B C D E** p.55

1.28 **A B C E** p.289

   D   autonomic hyperreflexia is associated with uncontrolled sympathetic discharge, i.e. tachycardia

1.29 **A D E** p.72

   B   there is initial hypercoagulability 3-4 weeks after stopping the Pill

   C   any cause of a low cardiac output increases the risk

1.30 **B D E** p.183
   A   it usually starts one week after a viral illness
   C   it is raised, usually being greater than 3 g/l

1.31 **A B C E** p.87
   C   such catheters should be connected to isolated (non-earthed monitors)
   D   current density is reduced

1.32 **A B C** p.107
   D   constant pressure generators; a decrease in patient compliance results in a fall in tidal volume
   E   2-3 ml/kg

1.33 **C** p.320

1.34 **B C D E** p.104
   A   ~50% of deaths associated with road traffic accidents

1.35 **A C** p.104
   B   cerebral acidosis may account for the recommencement of respiration

1.36 **B D** p.283
   A   autosomal dominant
   C   the heterozygous form provides some protection against falciparum malaria
   E   usually presents within the first year of life

1.37 **B D E** p.110
   A   1846
   C   1951

1.38 **C D** p.123
   A   1.15%
   B   enflurane, not isoflurane, causes such activity
   E   halothane is stored with thymol as a stabiliser

1.39 **B** p.148
   B   nitrous oxide supports combustion

1.40 **B C E** p.292
   A   it is bactericidal in 15 minutes but requires 3 hours to kill spores, and is therefore disinfection rather than sterilization
   D   high pressure and a temperature of ~130°C are required

1.41 **B C E** p.299
   A   radiated heat is lost

1.42 A B C p.302
   E rarely, an acute attack may provide short term immunity but active
      immunisation is generally required

1.43 B E p.283
   A adequate hydration is essential
   B because they have splenic dysfunction
   D an increased FIO_2 is required

1.44 B C D pp.9, 231

1.45 A C D p.229
   B pancuronium is an potential initiator of acute attacks
   E acute intermittent porphyria and variegate porphyria provide potential
      anaesthetic problems

1.46 A B p.183
   C presenting signs in the legs are classically upper motor neurone
   D the diagnosis is based on clinical findings and EMG studies

1.47 A B p.257
   E fine inspiratory crackles

1.48 A B E p.311
   C hypertension
   D hyperthermia

1.49 B D p.323
   A *Streptococcus viridans* is the most common causative agent
   C antibiotics are usually required intravenously for six weeks
   E it may have to be treated with valve replacement in the acute illness,
      although the mortality rate is high

1.50 A p.314
   B the tube is usually not changed for the first week
   C <20 mmHg
   E sedative premedicants should be avoided if the airway is compromised,
      antisialogogues may prevent expectoration of secretions in those with
      poor respiratory function

1.51 A B C D p.320
   E pulmonary oedema may occur

1.52 C D p.107
   A, B, E cardiovascular stability, low mean airway pressures, and use
            when there is a disrupted airway are proposed advantages

1.53   A C D E p.323
B   seronegative arthropathies are associated

1.54   A B E p.334
C   hypokalaemic alkalosis
D   intraocular pressure is likely to be elevated

1.55   B C E p.126
A   the agent must be specified before it can be measured
D   it is rapid
E   this is used in the Drager Narcotest (a historically interesting system)

1.56   A D E p.9
B   the murmur is described as millwheel
C   the end expiratory CO_2 falls acutely

1.57   C D E p.174
A   they tend to be low birth weight and premature
B   term babies that are at least one month old may be suitable for daycase care
C   a laryngeal mask airway may be used provided the hernia is not strangulated

1.58   A B C p.31
E   it is predominantly a test of the intrinsic pathway and is therefore very sensitive to the effect of heparin

1.59   B C p.34
A   it shifts to the left
D   hypoalbuminaemia results unless every transfused unit is whole blood

1.60   B C D E p.63
A   it reflects blood volume but is a measure of 'preload'

1.61   B C p. 98
A   investigation is warranted if there is no clear cause
D   hyponatraemia is associated with convulsions
E   hyperpyrexia is associated with convulsions

1.62   A B C p.63
D   Allen's test is neither sensitive nor specific and is therefore unlikely to reduce the risk of complications

1.63   A B C p.34
D   up to 6 units can be predonated
E   blood salvage is particularly useful in vascular and cardiac surgery

1.64 C E p.63
A   cardiac index = cardiac output/body surface area
D   SVR is a derived figure

1.65 B D E p.84
A   hyoscine causes confusion in the elderly

1.66 A B C D E p.114

1.67 B C D p.136
A   the posterior third of the tongue and the oropharynx are supplied by
    the glossopharyngeal nerve
E   second division (maxillary) of the trigeminal nerve

1.68 A C E p.148
D   saline should be used; nitrous oxide supports combustion

1.69 A C D E p.167
E   edrophonium may precipitate a cholinergic crisis

1.70 B C E p.22
A   a chest X-ray during an acute attack may show abnormal signs, but is
    not indicative of the severity of the attack

1.71 A B C D E p.179

1.72 A B D p.112
E   humidity is temperature and pressure dependent

1.73 D E p.114
C   prophylactic use may reduce the incidence/severity of acute episodes

1.74 A B D E p.120

1.75 B E p.152
A   free drug concentrations are increased due to hypoalbuminaemia
B   due to associated hypersplenism
C   metabolism is reduced
D   those with abnormal liver function often have reduced biliary excretion
E   FRC is reduced in the presence of ascites

1.76 A D E p.271
B   eye opening is assessed on a four-point scale
C   the minimum score is 3
D   this is a guideline figure for the need for ventilation

1.77 A E p.152
B solutions containing sodium or lactate should be avoided
C metabolic alkalosis
D lactulose is given to trap gut ammonia and reduce the risk of an encephalopathy developing

1.78 A B C E p.235
D eclamptic convulsions result from cerebral vasospasm

1.79 C D E p.271
A it is used to assess neonatal wellbeing at birth
B scores range from 0-2 for each of five variables; the maximum score is 10

1.80 B C D p.238
A umbilical vessels constrict in high O_2 concentrations
E increased acetylcholine levels following neostigmine administration may increase uterine tone

1.81 A B D E p.129
C the problems are maximal at birth

1.82 C D E p.241
A aspiration may occur during regional anaesthesia
B this is a relative contraindication

1.83 A B D p.186

1.84 C D E p.186
A hypothermia
B hypocalcaemia

1.85 A D p.78
B thiazide diuretics

1.86 A D E p.78
E β-blockade may mask the signs of hypoglycaemia

1.87 A C D E p.22
B an excessive decrease in pulse pressure occurs with significant pulsus paradoxus

1.88   A B D p.167
   A   as there is a risk of trauma to the superior vena cava during thymectomy
   C   patients are best rendered slightly myasthenic by reducing the dose of anticholinesterase preoperatively
   E   weakness improves with rest

1.89   ALL FALSE p.22
   A   a volume controlled ventilator will ensure an adequate tidal volume is delivered even if the respiratory compliance falls
   B   the expiratory phase should be prolonged
   D   theophylline metabolism may be reduced

1.90   C D E p.19
   B   the alveolar oedema is protein rich

ANSWERS TO PAPER TWO

The correct stems appear in bold
References refer to page numbers in *Key Topics in Anaesthesia* second edition

2.1 **A D** p.117
   B stimulation of the carotid sinus causes hypotension and bradycardia
   C hypercarbia
   E this will give a falsely low reading

2.2 **B** p.194
   A Cushing's syndrome and hypothyroidism, for example, also cause it
   C up to 5%
   D type II diabetes mellitus
   E it is increased

2.3 **B E** p.169
   A autosomal dominant
   C male:female incidence = 1:1

2.4 **B D E** p.197
   C hypercarbia is associated with a rise in intraocular pressure

2.5 **A C D** p.161
   B xenon and nitrous oxide are very different molecules from isoflurane
   E although the spinal cord shows decreased conduction the peripheral
      receptors are not affected

2.6 **A D E** p.225
   B V is proportional to T (constant pressure)
   C it is at the working temperature and pressure

2.7 **A D E** p.220
   C a number of agents may be used including morphine

2.8 **D E** p.66
   A the tetralogy includes a VSD
   B it is a cyanotic form of heart disease
   C it causes polycaethaemia as a response to hypoxia

2.9 **B D** p.191
   A blue cylinders with blue shoulders
   C nitrous oxide is more soluble in blood than nitrogen
   E it augments the respiratory depression of thiopentone

2.10 **A B D** p.207

C a magnet placed over the control box of some but not all pacemakers will convert them to a fixed pacing mode

E bipolar diathermy is safer

2.11 **B C E** p.167

A congenital myasthenia gravis is rare

D the female:male incidence is 3:2

E such as rheumatoid arthritis, pernicious anaemia, or thyrotoxicosis

2.12 **ALL FALSE** p.96

A intubation is best performed under deep volatile anaesthesia

B the child prefers to sit and drool as they cannot swallow saliva

C ampicillin and chloramphenicol are the best bet blind antibiotics

D adult epiglottitis also occurs

2.13 **B C D** p.201

A it may occur perioperatively during non fracture surgery

2.14 **C D** p.16

A the saturation may be normal even in the face of severe anaemia

E a normal haemoglobin for a 3-month old infant is 9-12 g/dl

2.15 **A C E** p.25

2.16 **C** p.1

A it usually results from an adrenocortical adenoma

B hypokalaemia

D adrenocortical deficiency is associated with hyperpigmentation

2.17 **B C D** p.132

A it is a carboxylated imadazole derivative

E pH ~5.0

2.18 **A B** p.4

C these are second line therapies

D in the absence of a palpable output cardiac compressions should be commenced regardless of the rhythm

E adrenaline is central to the treatment of severe reactions and should be administered early

2.19 **D E** p.37

A there must be no ventilatory effort

B >35°C

C an EEG is not required in the UK

2.20 D p.40

A formulae are only guides and considerably more fluid may be required

B analgesic requirements are high

E blood is often required

2.21 C D E p.55

A 80/minute

B over the lower half of the sternum

2.22 A p.44

B it is stored as a vapour

C it produces a fall in CSF pH

D it acts directly on the vessel wall to produce vasodilatation

E its effects are mediated via changes in CSF hydrogen ion concentration

2.23 A D p.72

C the association is with microvascular disease, not DVT

2.24 B D p.75

A the operating dentist is prohibited from also administering the general anaesthetic

C relative analgesia = 10-50% N_2O in O_2

E 24 hours

2.25 A B D p.203

C fibroplasia occurs behind the ocular lens

E it is attracted into a magnetic field

2.26 A B C E p.63

2.27 B C E p.63

A 89% of detectable ischaemic episodes

2.28 A C E p.69

B day surgery is acceptable from the age of 6 months

C patients should not drive within 24 hours

E whilst some ASA III patients with stable disease may be suitable for day surgery, those who are ASA IV are certainly not

2.29 B E p.84

A FRC and RV are both reduced

C closing volume exceeds FRC in the supine position from the age of 45

2.30 B C D E p.98

A the prevalence is 1:200 of the general population

2.31 C D p.112

A they are passive
B best performance = 33°C and 70% humidity

2.32 ALL FALSE p.114

A 100% O_2
B the minute ventilation should be increased to control the $PaCO_2$
C the initial dose of dantrolene is 1 mg/kg
D mannitol is often given E clotting may be abnormal

2.33 A B D E p.117

C the plasma volume is usually reduced

2.34 A B D p.120

2.35 C D E p.129

A mainly in males
B HLA B27

2.36 B C D p.146

2.37 B D pp.21, 126

A pink
C it is often found as a contaminant and levels of nitrogen dioxide must be measured in the breathing system
E up to a maximum of 20 parts per million

2.38 C E p.155

A 20% is metabolised
B halothane metabolism is usually oxidative

2.39 C E p.235

A 10% of pregnancies
D the triad, all features of which are not essential for diagnosis, consists of hypertension, proteinuria, and oedema

2.40 C p.271

A acute physiology and chronic health evaluation
B it is a tool to compare different units not patients
E the worst values in the first 24 hours

2.41 A B E p.52

2.42　A　p.261
　　　 B　lipid insoluble drugs are predominantly eliminated by the kidney
　　　 C　it alters binding site structure or configuration
　　　 D　hypervolaemia is more likely
　　　 E　metabolic acidosis

2.43　B C D E p.49
　　　 A　lignocaine is used to treat ventricular arrhythmias
　　　 B　may be used to treat atrial and ventricular arrhythmias

2.44　A B D p.276
　　　 C　sedation scores are multifactorial
　　　 E　postoperative patients always require analgesia. Analgesic techniques
　　　　　 reduce sedation requirements

2.45　A C D p.248
　　　 B　peaks at 32 weeks
　　　 E　it takes no account of aorto-caval compression

2.46　A B D E p.238
　　　 C　folate may reduce the incidence of neural tube defects

2.47　A B p.241
　　　 C　FRC is reduced and preoxygenation is thus achieved more rapidly.
　　　　　 Three vital capacity breaths of 100% O_2 may be sufficient
　　　 E　the 1 minute Apgar score is reduced by comparison with regional
　　　　　 techniques

2.48　A B p.241

2.49　B C E p.186
　　　 A　it binds to the postsynaptic membrane
　　　 D　there is a rise in oesophageal sphincter tone

2.50　C D p.186
　　　 A　the strength of the 4th twitch is decreased more than that of the 1st
　　　　　 twitch
　　　 B　50 Hz for 5 seconds

2.51　A B C D p.90

2.52　C D E p.78
　　　 A　2%
　　　 B　patients usually have some insulin function

2.53 B C E p.78

D   there is a reduced heart rate response to a Valsalva manoeuvre

2.54 B E p.100

A   machines that require an electrical supply may not function if disconnected

B   they should not be left attached to an anaesthetic machine

C   it should be calibrated as part of the machine check

D   -500 mmHg is required

2.55 B C p.19

A   pulmonary artery wedge pressure may be low or normal

D   low respiratory compliance

E   hypoxia is a more consistent finding

2.56 C E p.16

A   right shift

B   an oximeter measures the % of haemoglobin that is saturated with oxygen, and is unaffected by anaemia

2.57 D p.259

A   0.9% sodium chloride solution

B   a nasogastric tube is passed and gastric lavage performed preoperatively

C   there is frequently a secondary gastritis which has no bearing on the timing of surgery

E   a rapid sequence induction with cricoid pressure is appropriate

2.58 A p.268

C   it contains only activated charcoal

D   it is discarded on the basis of weight

E   it is not widely used because it does not scavenge N_2O

2.59 A B C p.285

E   the sympathetic cardiac accelerator fibres which arise from T_1/T_2 down to T_5 must all be blocked to produce a bradycardia

2.60 A E p.44

C   warm, bounding pulse peripheries

D   mydriasis

2.61 A D p.87

B   tachycardia

B   lower frequency is used for coagulation

E   it should never be used within 25 centimetres of a flammable anaesthetic source

2.62 A E p.93

B   24 hour urinary urea and creatinine collections help estimate nitrogen requirements but are no measure of malnutrition

2.63 A C D p.136

B, E   such patients should be protected from the stress and pressor response of an awake intubation

2.64 A B C E p.210

A   3 ml/kg/min for an adult, 6 ml/kg/min for an infant

2.65 B D E p.223

A   adrenal medulla

C   90% are benign

2.66 A B D E p.264

C   it falls with or without muscle relaxation

2.67 A D p.143

B   up to 75%

C   this tends to improve flow

E   it occurs mainly in diastole when myocardial wall tension is less

2.68 B C p.132

A   1% solution

D   more respiratory depression than thiopentone

E   more methohexitone than thiopentone is non-ionised and thus able to cross the blood-brain barrier

2.69 A B C p.107

D   120-6000 c.p.m.

E   expiration is active

2.70 A B E p.81

D   acidosis

2.71 A p.210

B   10% of the adult number of alveolae at birth

C   more compliant

D   there is no expiratory pause

E   there is an increased V:Q mismatch

2.72 B C E p.210
A hypoxaemic
D cardiac output is increased by increasing heart rate and not the stroke volume

2.73 C E p.294
A ADH levels rise
B prolactin levels rise
D adrenaline release predominates

2.74 A B D p.308
C a minimum FIO_2 of 0.5
E PEEP increases pulmonary vascular resistance and is thus not usually of benefit

2.75 A B C D p.266
E the anaemia is usually normochromic and normocytic

2.76 E p.283
A there is a normal life expectancy
D the haemoglobin is usually >11 g/dl

2.77 A D E p.66
B although associated with Turners syndrome it is commoner in males
C it is usually distal to the origin of the left subclavian artery

2.78 C D p.292
A it kills neither
B boiling is an example of disinfection
E 10% sodium hypochlorite is required following hepatitis B contamination

2.79 C E p.297
B a low capacity allows the rapid development of a high negative pressure
D negative pressure is displayed in an anticlockwise direction

2.80 D E p.299
A it is affected by respiratory gases in the unintubated patient and risks nasopharyngeal mucosal damage
B resistance changes non-linearly with temperature
C changes in temperature affect the voltage produced

2.81 A B E p.302
C the severity of symptoms increases for 2-3 days
D *Clostridium tetani* is difficult to grow in culture

2.82 B C D p.231
A the medial aspect is at greater risk

2.83 A E p.158
B MRI interferes with the conduction of electricity and therefore oximetry
C it is very claustrophobic and noisy and not well tolerated by young children
D it may take up to one hour to perform an MRI investigation

2.84 B C p.183
A heat is more likely to cause an exacerbation
E regional anaesthesia has not been shown to worsen symptoms but is likely to be blamed in the event of any postoperative deterioration

2.85 C p.229

2.86 A B D E p.311
C acute hypocalcaemia may occur

2.87 B C D p.323
A presystolic accentuation is only possible if the patient is in sinus rhythm
E pulmonary vasoconstriction should be avoided

2.88 E p.327
A renal perfusion is reduced regardless of the level of cross clamping
B myocardial strain is most likely at cross clamping
C an adequate perfusion pressure is essential before these measures
D there is washback of acidotic blood which also causes a fall in blood pressure

2.89 A C D p.9
B tachycardia is more likely
E hypotension

2.90 A C D p.28
B the risk is 0.6%

ANSWERS TO PAPER THREE

The correct stems appear in bold
References refer to page numbers in *Key Topics in Anaesthesia* second edition

3.1   **C D E** p.28
A   the filter found in blood giving sets is usually between 180 and 200 μm
B   microaggregates occur particularly from white cells

3.2   **C E** p.31
B   although the intrinsic pathway does contain factor X which is vitamin K dependent it is affected much later than the extrinsic pathway which includes Factor VII
D   the normal result is 39-42 seconds

3.3   **A B C E** p.47
B   enterochromaffin cells are also known as argentiffan cells
D   the primary is usually in the small bowel

3.4   **B** p.143
A   the resting ECG is often normal, an exercise ECG is required
C   coronary steal only occurs at high MACs
D   a high preload causes a high LVEDV which increases oxygen demand
E   this is normal when ischaemic heart disease is present unless a recent MI has occurred

3.5   **A B D E** p.266
C   there is no association with focal epilepsy

3.6   **B C D E** p.283
A   acidosis not alkalosis will precipitate sickling

3.7   **A B E** p.289
A   the massive sympathetic discharge may cause a CVA
C   residual volume increases
D   although advisable it is not considered mandatory in the UK

3.8   **C** p.299
A   the risk is of ventricular fibrillation below 28°C
B   the level of consciousness decreases below 30°C
D   urine output is preserved as ADH secretion is suppressed
E   MAC falls by 7% per degree in temperature

3.9   C D E p.302
- A   is more common in men (2.5:1)
- B   alters inhibitory synaptic function

3.10   B C D E p.231
- A   chest compliance falls
- D   this may be related to venous congestion

3.11   B C p.229
- A   faecal porphyrins are found (aminolaevulinic acid is found in those with acute intermittent porphyria)
- D   the deficiency is of protoporphyrinogen oxidase
- E   they are more common in South Africa

3.12   B C D p.257
- A   the capillary permeability is increased
- E   the usual lymphatic drainage is 500 ml per day

3.13   C p.66
- A   patients with abnormal cardiac anatomy should receive antibiotics
- B   this would increase left to right shunt and worsen cyanosis
- D   it is faster as blood carrying the induction agent reaches the brain quicker
- E   the risk is increased with a right to left shunt

3.14   A C D E p.311
- A   the superior vena cava may be obstructed by a retrosternal goitre
- C   collapse of the trachea may occur following removal of the gland

3.15   B C E p.158
- A   it is at 50 Gauss
- D   it produces a magnetic field that is 10 000 to 20 000 times stronger than the earth's

3.16   B C E p.314
- A   this is a late complication
- C   this may occur on sudden correction of the respiratory acidosis caused by the airway obstruction
- D   a late complication

3.17   C E p.320
- A   it is a 1.5% solution and is iso-osmotic
- B   it is a poor electrical conductor thus allowing diathermy to be used
- D   is absorbed at a rate of approximately 20 ml/min

3.18 A D p.334

B butyrophenones work at the chemoreceptor trigger zone which has doperminergic receptors

D they act at the vomiting centre that lies within the blood-brain barrier

E etomidate causes more postoperative emesis than other induction agents

3.19 C D E p.7

A the 'window' period refers to the development of antibodies and not to the development of the full syndrome

B T helper cells are preferentially affected /

3.20 A C D p.9

B nitrous oxide is 34 times more soluble

E the left lateral head down position is used

3.21 C E p.28

A blood is stored at 4°C

B a minimum of 70% of cells should be viable 24 hours after transfusion

D this gives a shelf life of 21 days

3.22 C D E p.31

A tests the extrinsic pathway

B the vitamin K dependent factors are II, VII and X

C factor VII is the first to decrease with warfarin

3.23 B C D E p.31

A Gram negative infections are more likely to precipitate DIC than Gram positive infections

3.24 B p.33

A whether a patient is ready to be weaned or not is multifactorial but if the PaO_2 is more than 8 kPa with an FiO_2 the patient may be weaned

C Synchronised Intermittent Mandatory Ventilation

D PEEP may be useful

E a tracheostomy usually makes weaning the patient easier as it decreases the work of breathing and enables a lighter level of sedation to be achieved when compared with a patient with an orotracheal tube

3.25 C D E p.308

3.26 **A B D** p.40

B the oxygen tension as measured by a blood gas analyser is normal but the total content is markedly decreased

C pulse oximeters are unable to differentiate haemoglobin that is carrying carbon monoxide rather than oxygen

E it has an affinity 250 times that of oxygen

3.27 **B D E** p.40

A the rise in potassium related to suxamethonium does not occur for several hours following a burn injury

B up to twice the dose of the non-depolarising muscle relaxant may be needed

C the peak is at 4 days

3.28 **A B** p.47

C fibrosis results in right sided cardiac valvular lesions but not pulmonary fibrosis

D this occurs with a phaeochromocytoma

E right sided lesions

3.29 **C D** p.194

A the body mass index is the weight (kg) divided by the square of the height (m) and morbid obesity is a BMI >35

B gastric residual volume is also increased

D cardiac index takes body surface area into account

E the dose should be reduced

3.30 **A B E** p.220

B the MEAC is the plasma level of opioid required by an individual to be adequately analgesed

C background infusions do not improve the quality of analgesia

D may be used in children as young as 5

3.31 **A E** p.225

B turbulent flow is likely if the Reynolds number is >2000

C when flow is laminar, viscosity not density affects the rate of flow

D the gap is tubular and is therefore likely to result in laminar flow

3.32 **B C E** p.169

A loss of the eyebrows is seen in hypothyroidism

D no facial rash is described

3.33 **A C D E** p.174

A 1 in 5000 live births versus 1 in 30 000

B this is the cause of gastroschiasis

3.34 B C D p.174

A the incidence varies between different units

E the mortality rate is approximately 50%

3.35 A E p.197

B lignocaine may be used to decrease the pressor response to laryngoscopy and thus prevent a rise in intraocular pressure

D ecothiopate drops are used to treat glaucoma

3.36 C D p.197

A a long 25 gauge needle is required

B 2 ml of lignocaine 2% is used

E the branches of the VIIth nerve to the eye also need to be blocked

3.37 A D E p.201

B data vary, but 2.5 hours is too long

C a metabolic acidosis

3.38 B C D E p.25

A Guedel's signs are not specific to ether

D MAC is reduced by sedative premedicants

3.39 A B D E p.1

A adrenal haemorrhage may cause an Addisonian picture

C hypoglycaemia is commonly found

3.40 B C D p.37

A the pupillary responses also test the parasympathetics

E the gag reflex does not test the 11th cranial nerve

3.41 A E p.55

B bretylium tosylate is used to treat resistant ventricular fibrillation

C adrenaline should be given every 2-3 minutes

D bicarbonate in the presence of hypoventilation will worsen intracellular acidosis and shift the oxygen dissociation curve to the left thus worsening tissue hypoxia

3.42 D p.66

A secundum is far more common than primum

B it has fixed splitting due to increased pulmonary blood flow

C if pulmonary blood pressure rises the murmur gets quieter

E it is repaired through the right atrium as this lies anteriorly

3.43   A B p.72
   D   aprotinin is used to prevent bradykinin release in the management of the carcinoid syndrome
   E   an increased FIO_2 has no effect in decreasing DVT

3.44   C D p.81
   B   the diving reflex results in vasoconstriction
   E   PEEP is generally used to improve gas exchange

3.45   B C p.132
   A   thiopentone is highly alkaline with a pH of 11
   B   this prevents atmospheric CO_2 from forming the insoluble free acid form
   D   reawakening occurs due to redistribution
   E   it is metabolised prior to excretion

3.46   A B C p.167
   D   it is not associated with primary hyperaldosteronism (Conn's syndrome)
   E   frontal bossing is seen in the homozygous form of β-thalassaemia

3.47   C E p.203
   A   capillary oxygen tension is measured
   B   low cardiac output with poor skin perfusion causes inaccuracy
   C   the skin heated to 44°C
   D   it has no particular benefits in burns patients

3.48   A E p.179
   B   the pressure is normally zero
   C   autoregulation normally occurs over the range 50-160 mmHg of mean arterial pressure
   D   it is not pressure dependent within the range of autoregulation

3.49   B D p.60
   A   this occurs due to atrial contraction but is not one of the quoted 'risk factors'
   C   this is a normal finding
   E   an ejection fraction of less than 40% suggests significant risk

3.50   C E p.63
   A   the cannula should be non-tapering
   B   it should be non-compliant to prevent damping
   D   the cuff width should be equal to 40% of the circumference of the patient's arm

3.51 B C E p.69
A identical preoperative assessment should occur
D the patient needs the same amount of care

3.52 A C D E p.98
B hypocalcaemia

3.53 B E p.84
A 30% loss
C cerebral oxygen consumption falls
D it falls by 1% per year after the age of 30

3.54 B D E p.112
A it is the actual mass of water vapour in a given volume of gas at a specified temperature and pressure (g/m^3)
C condensation occurs when a gas becomes fully saturated: this is the dew point
D the latent heat of vaporisation
E as humidity increases

3.55 A B D p.112
C the baffle removes large droplets so that only small droplets are inhaled
E the risk is increased

3.56 E p.114
A it rises by 2°C per hour
B the early signs are tachycardia, increased CO_2 production and muscle rigidity
C there is no correlation
D hyperkalaemia

3.57 A C D p.114
B it shows autosomal dominant inheritance with impaired penetrance
E the gene locus is on the long arm of chromosome 19

3.58 A B C D p.117
D the blood pressure may be low, normal or elevated
E it is seen with both of these conditions

3.59 A B D E p.155
C hepatic blood supply is a low pressure system and thus is readily affected by mechanical pressure changes (e.g. surgical retraction)

3.60 **A B** p.117
    D alfentanil or fentanyl have a more rapid effect
    E this is performed at laryngoscopy!

3.61 **A C** p.120
    B autoregulation occurs down to a MAP of 50 mmHg
    D this is lost below 35 mmHg
    E direct acting vasodilators are better

3.62 **A C D** p.129
    B it is the meiotic non-dysjunctional form that is related to maternal age
    E 50%

3.63 **D** p.129
    A X-linked
    B the bleeding time is normal (the direct acting vasodilators are better intrinsic clotting pathways are affected)
    C levels approaching 100% of normal should be achieved
    E epidurals are contraindicated

3.64 **A D E** p.164
    C a maximum of 3 litres should be insufflated
    D this procedure can be performed under local anaesthesia
    E the combination of Trendelenburg and a raised intra-abdominal pressure make airway protection with a tracheal tube advisable

3.65 **A B C E** p.146
    A radiotherapy may be given preoperatively
    D there is no contraindication and a dry operative field may be of benefit

3.66 **A D** p.152
    B the bleeding time is not dependent on hepatic clotting factors
    C the albumin is more specific

3.67 **A B D E** p.280
    C 20-30% develop MODS

3.68 **B E** p.37
    A they do not need to be performed simultaneously
    C only one set is needed by law
    D the doctors must both be 5 years post-registration

3.69 **A C D E** p.40
    B the rule of nines, each leg is 2 x 9% = 18%
    E as plasma proteins are lost through the burn

3.70 A B D E p.47
C sympathomimetics may stimulate the further release of vasodilators
from the tumour

3.71 D p.245
A T_{10} - L_1
B 40 - 150 Hz
C 30%
E this is the point at which neonatal respiratory depression will be
maximal

3.72 A B C D p.19
B when partially reduced leads to the formation of toxic free radicals
E asthma alone is unlikely to result in ARDS

3.73 A B p.235
B related to hepatic congestion
D not in the initial uncomplicated pre-eclamptic
E hyperreflexia

3.74 B C p.235
C due to laryngeal oedema
D magnesium sulphate potentiates non-depolarising relaxants
E in a patient with a potential bleeding diathesis the subclavian approach
to a central vein is contraindicated

3.75 A C p.52
B the pump prime is approximately 2 litres but it is not usual to use blood
except in small children
D it is over efficient and may necessitate the addition of CO_2 to the
returning blood
E 3 mg/kg (300 units/kg) is the normal dose of heparin

3.76 A E p.60
B coronary perfusion predominantly occurs during diastole, with
diastolic pressure therefore more important than systolic
C left ventricular end diastolic pressure
D it is the pressure rather than the volume
E this affects the oxygen content of the blood

3.77 B C D p.268
A,E 5% sodium hydroxide, 90% calcium hydroxide, 1% potassium
hydroxide plus silicates and an indicator

3.78 **B E** p.261

    A it is usually normochromic and normocytic

    B related to uraemia

    D it is normally be transfused at this time

3.79 **C** p.261

    A dialysis is usually performed prior to transplantation and the potassium is not normally elevated

    B Hartmann's solution contains lactate and is avoided

    D these lines are not always required - the 'norm' for different centres varies

    E vasopressors may reduce renal perfusion

3.80 **A C E** p.271

    B age >70 years

    D myocardial infarction within the last 6 months

3.81 **B C D** p.271

    A six more variables are used than in APACHE II

    E resource utilisation is not the aim

3.82 **C D** p.152

    B spironolactone, a potassium preserving diuretic, is the drug of choice

    E it increases intra-abdominal pressure and therefore reduces FRC

3.83 **D E** p.276

    A morphine-6-glucuronide

    B norpethidine will accumulate in renal dysfunction

    D the problem is that the half life of its metabolite is 96 hours

3.84 **A** p.253

    B shorter times are acceptable in children

    C both sensitivity and specificity should be high, approaching 100%

    D 70%

    E this is not recommended

3.85 **A** p.245

    B the addition of opioids to local anaesthetics reduces the incidence of assisted delivery

    C the block needs to reach T_{1-4} to cause a bradycardia

    D 70%

    E the overall dural tap rate of a unit should be less than 1%

3.86 A D E p.248

    B gastric emptying is delayed due to increased progesterone, decreased motilin and mechanical displacement

    C gastrin levels are elevated producing hyperacidity

    D opinion differs over when to start taking precautions, but most seem agreed upon the 18th week

3.87 A D E p.194

    B 80% of the normal mg/kg dose is recommended

    E is the technique of choice if possible

3.88 E p.238

    A glycopyrrolate is preferred as it does not cross the placenta

    B the hyperventilation should match her norm

    D this should be used from the 20th week

3.89 A D p.186

    C less than 30 suggests homozygous, 40-60 heterozygous and >70 homozygous - normal

    E a prolonged block may be anticipated

3.90 A B D p.78

    A e.g. surgery to control infection

    B during the acute management normal saline is used until the blood sugar has fallen to 10 mmol/l at which point 5% glucose is substituted

    C total body stores are depleted despite the finding of a high extracellular potassium

    E the acidosis is of a metabolic origin and rarely requires ventilatory support

ANSWERS TO PAPER FOUR

The correct stems appear in bold
References refer to page numbers in *Key Topics in Anaesthesia* second edition

4.1   **C D** p.98
A   anticonvulsants should be continued up to and including the day of surgery
C,D   both agents may lower the seizure threshold

4.2   **A B C E** p.16
D   hypersplenism may cause anaemia

4.3   **C D** p.22
B   disease severity is best assessed by spirometry
E   an elevated $PaCO_2$ is a late sign during a severe asthma attack and is not normal

4.4   **B C E** p.191
A   it is a vapour at room temperature

4.5   **A B D** p.167
C   this is a cholinergic crisis
E   10%

4.6   **A C D** p.34
E   transmission of the Epstein-Barr virus may occur but this does not cause hand, foot and mouth disease

4.7   **A D E** p.323
B   aortic stenosis causes concentric left ventricular hypertrophy
C   the murmur is pan-systolic

4.8   **A C** p.289
B   autonomic hyperreflexia is decreased by spinal anaesthesia
E   airway secretions are readily retained and a drying agent may well be needed; there is no contraindication to the use of an antisialagogue

4.9   **D** p.104
A,B   both will increase ICP and thus produce a fall in cerebral perfusion
C   draining CSF may reduce ICP but is a dangerous manoeuvre under these circumstances as it risks cerebral herniation and coning
E   thiopentone will reduce cerebral O_2 demand but any associated fall in mean arterial pressure will result in a fall in cerebral perfusion

4.10   A C p.207
B   patients with bifasicular block that is symptomatic require pacing preoperatively
D,E   these are unlikely to progress to cardiovascularly unstable rhythms

4.11   B D E p.169
C   hyperkalaemia

4.12   C E p.210
A   high pulse rate and low blood pressure
B   narrowest at the level of the cricoid ($C_{3/4}$)
D   more sensitive to the respiratory depressant effects of opioids

4.13   C D p.84
A   vascular compliance decreases
B   baroreceptor sensitivity increases
E   total body water is decreased

4.14   A D p.259
B   ~1:350
C   ~85% are males
E   unknown aetiology

4.15   C D E p.268
A   30 mm male

4.16   B C E p.285
A   long term mortality in this group of patients is the same with general or spinal anaesthesia
D   the contraindication is relative

4.17   C D E p.81
A   it is more likely to occur in children
B   marked bradycardia

4.18   A D E p.223
A   as this will tend to increase blood pressure
B   patients usually have a low CVP and require fluid resuscitation
C   it sensitises the myocardium to the high circulating catecholamines

4.19   B C E p.264
A   the response to hypoxia is more greatly depressed

4.20 B C E p.207

A the first letter refers to the paced chamber

D any necessary DC shocks should ideally be given at 90° to the pacing wire

4.21 D E p.155

A 25% of cardiac output

B 20% of inspired halothane is metabolised

4.22 A B E p.66

C it is performed very early to ensure some blood mixing occurs between the otherwise parallel, independent circulations

4.23 C D p.225

A degrees Kelvin

B the Newton is a unit of force

E seven basic units

4.24 A C D pp.78, 72, 117

C there is an increased risk of DVT/PE. Rebound hypercoagulability occurs about four weeks after stopping the Pill, six should thus elapse

D anticoagulation should be converted to heparin which is more easily controlled in the short term

4.25 B C p.220

A when in control of their own analgesia most patients will accept a basal degree of pain

E loading should be employed to provide adequate analgesia before handing over control of analgesic dosing to the patient. This is important for patient confidence

4.26 C p.174

A 50% have associated abnormalities

B polyhydramnios

D intubation whilst the neonate is breathing spontaneously avoids positive pressure ventilation and the risk of gastric distension

4.27 A B D E p.174

C the lung is usually hypoplastic

E bowel distension will worsen pulmonary function

4.28 A E p.280

B it is found in smooth muscles

C has a half life of just a few seconds

D it increases intracellular cyclic guanosine monophosphate

4.29   B C D p.197
A   nitrous oxide causes a rise in IOP if there is gas in the eye

4.30   A B C E p.201

4.31   A B D E p.201
C   hypotensive anaesthesia may reduce blood loss

4.32   E p.96
A   it is usually caused by Haemophilus influenzae type B
B   the peak incidence is in children aged 2-5 years
C   the neck X-ray is often unnecessary and may endanger the child if they are sent to the X-ray department without someone skilled in paediatric intubation
D   the pain of an intramuscular injection may precipitate crying and complete respiratory obstruction. Oral premeds cannot be swallowed

4.33   A B C D E p.4

4.34   A B p.60
C   M mode is better for valve structure
D   the function of hypokinetic areas (and therefore of the heart generally) is likely to worsen during ischaemia
E   a MUGA scan is relatively non-invasive

4.35   B D p.299
C   0.2 g in force is positive

4.36   ALL FALSE p.140
A   assessment is performed seated in front of a patient at the same height
B   assessment is purely visual without the aid of instruments
C   this is class 1
D   the grading is a predictor of the findings at laryngoscopy

4.37   A B E p.93
C   70 g of protein per day
D   lactase, required for the metabolism of lactose, is frequently deficient in the malnourished, postoperative patient

4.38   A B D E p.78

4.39 **B** p.16

    A volume of oxygen in a known volume of blood i.e. ml/dl

    C oxygen content x cardiac output

    D dissolved oxygen = 0.0225 ml x PaO_2 (kPa)

    E haemoglobin of ~10 g/dl provides optimum oxygen delivery

4.40 **C E** p.331

    A if lung compliance decreases when a pressure generator is used, the tidal volume will fall

    B although the flow is constant, the pressure will vary with lung compliance

    D this ventilator uses the energy of the compressed gases as its power source

4.41 **A E** p.129

    B it may be associated with arachnodactyly

    C upward displacement of the lens

    D there may be difficulty with intubation, cardiac and respiratory complications

4.42 **B C D E** p.164

    A should not usually exceed 30 cmH_2O

    E if large amounts of CO_2 are absorbed

4.43 **A D E** p.25

    B smooth muscle lower oesophageal contractions continue even in the presence of neuromuscular blockade

4.44 **A C E** p.314

    B is often performed on the intensive care unit

    D should not be sited immediately below the cricoid as this may increase the incidence of late stricture

4.45 **A C D E** p.44

    B it is measured indirectly via a change in hydrogen ion concentration

4.46 **A B D** p.40

    C pulse oximeters are currently unable to detect differences in haemoglobin species

    E hyperbaric oxygen therapy is used for severe carbon monoxide poisoning

4.47 **A B C D E** p.72

4.48   A E p.123
B a low blood gas solubility will ensure rapid onset and wake-up
C the ideal agent will be excreted unchanged
D a boiling point higher than room temperature is desirable

4.49   A B C p.123
D 20% metabolised
E 0.01% thymol

4.50   B D E p.132
A the limb should be kept warm and well perfused
E vasodilatation should be encouraged

4.51   B D p.140
A this is a classification of antiarrhythmic agents
C a thyromental distance of <6.5 cm
E increased anterior depth of the mandible results in difficulty

4.52   B D p.55
A,B   this is recommended for witnessed or monitored arrests, VT and
      torsade de pointes
C   200 J
E   this is no longer recommended

4.53   C D p.148
A laser energy is monochromatic
B far infra-red (10 600 nm)
E penetrates up to a depth of 200 mm

4.54   A C p.179
B,E   this is a sign of meningism

4.55   B C D p.136
A Krause's method is for a superior laryngeal nerve block
E this will anaesthetise the subglottic region

4.56   B E p.203
C a fuel cell does not require a voltage
D oxygen combines with electrons at the cathode

4.57   A B C D E p.203
C tricuspid incompetence produces a pulsatile venous bed and leads to an
   underestimation of the haemoglobin saturation

4.58 B p.292

A it has high antiviral activity
D 2% gluteraldehyde is recommended
E it is a method of disinfection

4.59 E p.299

A highest at 1500 hrs
B heat is also produced by metabolism and is gained from food intake
C anterior thalamus
D absolute zero is zero degrees Kelvin (K)

4.60 B D E p.34

A 46.5% of the population
C 3% of the population

4.61 B D p.299

A it causes a left shift in the oxygen dissociation curve
C it is associated with hyperglycaemia
E 'J' waves occur with hypothermia

4.62 B D E p.297

A surgical requirement is for a high displacement
C the British standard requires the generation of -400 mmHg

4.63 E p.280

A 'blind' antibiotic therapy may be required if the patient is severely ill
B a longer inspiratory time is aiming to decrease the peak airway pressures
C this is the acceptance of a raised arterial carbon dioxide provided that marked systemic acidosis does not occur
D glutamine is given to protect gastrointestinal function

4.64 C p.251

4.65 D p.183

A diagnosis is a clinical one supported by MRI findings
B equal sex incidence
C commonest between 20 and 40 years

4.66 B pp.183, 167

D upper motor neurone and sensory deficits

4.67 B C p.186

A hyperkalaemia
E associated with hypokalaemia

4.68 A C E p.229
B motor neuropathy and seizures are not uncommon

4.69 C E p.327
A it is the ipsilateral hemisphere which is perfused by the Circle of Willis
B <50 mmHg

4.70 B E p.334
A inside the blood brain barrier
C acetylcholine is the predominant neurotransmitter
D the chemoreceptor trigger zone lies in the lateral wall of the ventricle

4.71 A B D p.320
C fluid overload is likely to be hypo-osmolar
E this implies sub-diaphragmatic intraperitoneal soiling and should not occur during an extraperitoneal procedure such as TURP

4.72 B p.323
C a slow rising low pressure pulse
E there is hypertrophy but dilation occurs with aortic regurgitation

4.73 A C D E p.7
B gloves need only be worn when there is a risk of contact with infected body fluids

4.74 A B D E p.9

4.75 A C D p.28
B osmotic fragility is increased
E clinically significant impairment of clotting occurs after one week

4.76 B D E p.31
A it measures the time taken to clot following a standardised incision
C >150 mg/100 ml

4.77 B D p.31
A <160 mg/100 ml
C >15 seconds
E the thrombin time is prolonged

4.78 B D E p.37
A a markedly elevated $PaCO_2$ may itself alter conscious state
C there must be no spontaneous respiration

4.79 B p.66
- A bypass is required to allow the right ventricle to be opened
- C it closes spontaneously in only 50%
- D small VSDs cause loud murmurs which get quieter if the right and left pressures equate
- E when there is a left to right shunt the pulmonary arteries increase in size

4.80 A C E p.40
- B circumferential burns of the neck necessitate early intubation
- D this amount of carboxyhaemoglobin will not by itself prevent adequate tissue oxygenation; a figure of 40% COHb is probably more appropriate

4.81 A C D p.60
- E clinical findings show a poor correlation

4.82 D E p.191
- A 105%
- B the pressure gauge provides no information about the cylinder contents until all the liquid has vaporised

4.83 B C p.123
- A it is a halogenated ether
- E desflurane requires a special vaporiser

4.84 A C D p.132
- B isotonic
- E it is primarily excreted in the urine

4.85 ALL FALSE p.4
- B volume loading is usually required
- C the anaesthetic should be withdrawn as soon as is practicable
- D adrenaline should be given early and intravenously

4.86 D p.1
- A it is a mineralocorticoid
- B it is secreted by the zona glomerulosa
- C it causes increased renal sodium reabsorption
- E renin is not converted to angiotensin

4.87 D p.216
- A 150-200% of the parenteral dose
- B the bioavailability is much reduced after swallowing
- C intercostal cryoanalgesia usually misses the posterior primary rami

4.88   **A B E** p.294
   C   there is salt retention at the kidney
   D   circulating free fatty acids are increased

4.89   **A C D E** p.304
   B   secretion retention is a problem if the FEV_1 <1.0 litre

4.90   **C D E** p.304
   A   the incidence is ~4.5% following pneumonectomy
   B   it is typically associated with an empyema